Hair

Editor

NEIL S. SADICK

DERMATOLOGIC CLINICS

www.derm.theclinics.com

Consulting Editor
BRUCE H. THIERS

July 2021 • Volume 39 • Number 3

ELSEVIER

1600 John F. Kennedy Boulevard • Suite 1800 • Philadelphia, Pennsylvania, 19103-2899

http://www.theclinics.com

DERMATOLOGIC CLINICS Volume 39, Number 3
July 2021 ISSN 0733-8635, ISBN-13: 978-0-323-79161-8

Editor: Lauren Boyle
Developmental Editor: Karen Justine Solomon

Dermatologic Clinics (ISSN 0733-8635) is published quarterly by Elsevier Inc., 360 Park Avenue South, New York, NY 10010-1710. Months of publication are January, April, July, and October. Business and editorial offices: 1600 John F. Kennedy Blvd., Suite 1800, Philadelphia, PA 19103-2899. Customer service office: 11830 Westline Drive, St. Louis, MO 63146. Periodicals postage paid at New York, NY, and additional mailing offices. Subscription prices are USD 416.00 per year for US individuals, USD 1,000.00 per year for US institutions, USD 456.00 per year for Canadian individuals, USD 1,055.00 per year for Canadian institutions, USD 510.00 per year for international individuals, USD 1,055.00 per year for international institutions, USD 100.00 per year for US students/residents, USD 100.00 per year for Canadian students/residents, and USD 240 per year for international students/residents. International air speed delivery is included in all *Clinics* subscription prices. All prices are subject to change without notice. **POSTMASTER:** Send address changes to *Dermatologic Clinics*, Elsevier Health Sciences Division, Subscription Customer Service, 3251 Riverport Lane, Maryland Heights, MO 63043. **Customer Service: 1-800-654-2452 (U.S. and Canada); 314-447-8871 (outside U.S. and Canada). Fax: 314-447-8029. E-mail: journalscustomerservice-usa@elsevier.com (for print support); journalsonlinesupport-usa@elsevier.com (for online support).**

Reprints. For copies of 100 or more, of articles in this publication, please contact the Commercial Reprints Department, Elsevier Inc., 360 Park Avenue South, New York, New York 10010-1710. Tel.: 212-633-3874; Fax: 212-633-3820; Email: reprints@elsevier.com.

The *Dermatologic Clinics* is covered in *MEDLINE/PubMed (Index Medicus)*, *Current Contents/Clinical Medicine*, *Excerpta Medica*, *Chemical Abstracts*, and *ISI/BIOMED*.

Contributors

CONSULTING EDITOR

BRUCE H. THIERS, MD
Professor and Chairman Emeritus, Department
of Dermatology and Dermatologic Surgery,
Medical University of South Carolina,
Charleston, South Carolina, USA

EDITOR

**NEIL S. SADICK, MD, FACP, FAACS, FACPh,
FAAD**
Clinical Professor, Department of
Dermatology, Weill Medical College of Cornell
University, New York, New York, USA; Faculty,
Department of Dermatology, University of
Minnesota, Minneapolis, Minnesota, USA;
Medical Director, Sadick Dermatology; Past
President of the AACS, ISDS

AUTHORS

GLYNIS ABLON, MD, FAAD
Associate Clinical Professor, UCLA
Dermatology, Manhattan Beach, California,
USA

SULEIMA ARRUDA, MD
Department of Dermatology, Weill Medical
College of Cornell University, New York, New
York, USA

MARC R. AVRAM, MD
Clinical Professor of Dermatology, Weill Cornell
Medical School, New York, New York, USA;
Private Practice

AWA BAKAYOKO, BA
Lewis Katz School of Medicine, Temple
University, Philadelphia, Pennsylvania,
USA

GRETCHEN BELLEFEUILLE, BS
Research Intern, Department of Dermatology,
University of Minnesota, Minneapolis,
Minnesota, USA

VALERIE D. CALLENDER, MD, FAAD
Callender Dermatology and Cosmetic Center,
Glenn Dale, Maryland, USA; Professor of
Dermatology, Howard University College of
Medicine, Washington, DC, USA

KRISTINA COLLINS, MD
Private Practice, Austin, Texas, USA

AMANDA EISINGER, DO
Pilaris, OnDERMAND Dermatology, New York,
New York, USA

RONDA S. FARAH, MD
Assistant Professor, Department of
Dermatology, University of Minnesota,
Minneapolis, Minnesota, USA

ADITYA K. GUPTA, MD, PhD
Professor, Division of Dermatology,
Department of Medicine, University of Toronto
School of Medicine, Toronto, Ontario, Canada;
Director, Mediprobe Research Inc, London,
Ontario, Canada

SPENCER D. HAWKINS, MD
Resident, Department of Dermatology,
University of Michigan, Ann Arbor, Michigan,
USA

MARIA HORDINSKY, MD
Professor and Chair, Department of
Dermatology, University of Minnesota,
Minneapolis, Minnesota, USA

JARED JAGDEO, MD, MS
Dermatology Service, VA New York Harbor
Healthcare System, Department of
Dermatology, SUNY Downstate Medical
Center, Brooklyn, New York, USA

NATALIE KASH, MD, FAAD
Program Faculty, Department of Dermatology,
Kansas City University-Graduate Medical
Education Consortium/Advanced
Dermatology and Cosmetic Surgery
Orlando Dermatology Program, Maitland,
Florida, USA

BISMA KHALID, MBBS, FCPS
Research Fellow, University of Minnesota,
Minneapolis, Minnesota, USA

ALANA KURTTI, BS
Rutgers Robert Wood Johnson Medical
School, Piscataway, New Jersey, USA;
Dermatology Service, VA New York
Harbor Healthcare System, Brooklyn,
New York, USA

CHRISTINA N. LAWSON, MD, FAAD
Dermatology Associates of Lancaster,
Lancaster, Pennsylvania, USA

ADAM LEAVITT, MD
Resident, Department of Dermatology,
University of Michigan, Ann Arbor, Michigan,
USA

MATT LEAVITT, DO, FAOCD
Chairman, Department of Dermatology,
Kansas City University-Graduate Medical
Education Consortium/Advanced Dermatology
and Cosmetic Surgery Orlando Dermatology
Program, Founder, Executive Chairman,
Advanced Dermatology and Cosmetic
Surgery, Maitland, Florida, USA; Assistant

Professor, University of Central Florida,
College of Medicine, Orlando, Florida, USA;
Executive Medical Advisor, Bosley Medical
Group, Maitland, Florida, USA

JAMES T. PATHOULAS, BA
Medical Student, Department of Dermatology,
University of Minnesota, Minneapolis,
Minnesota, USA

JEFFREY A. RAPAPORT, MD
Director, Cosmetic Skin and Surgery Center,
Englewood Cliffs, New Jersey, USA

ORA RAYMOND, BA
Research Intern, Department of Dermatology,
University of Minnesota, Minneapolis,
Minnesota, USA

HELEN J. RENAUD, PhD
Research Associate, Mediprobe Research Inc,
London, Ontario, Canada

RAHIL B. ROOPANI, MD
Fellow, Hair Restoration Surgery Program,
Leavitt Medical Associates, Maitland, Florida,
USA

PAUL T. ROSE, MD, FAAD, FISHRS, JD
Miami Skin and Hair Institute, Coral Gables,
Florida, USA

**NEIL S. SADICK, MD, FACP, FAACS, FACPh,
FAAD**
Clinical Professor, Department of
Dermatology, Weill Medical College of Cornell
University, New York, New York, USA; Faculty,
Department of Dermatology, University of
Minnesota, Minneapolis, Minnesota, USA;
Medical Director, Sadick Dermatology; Past
President of the AACS, ISDS

KUMAR SUKHDEO, MD, PhD
Pilaris, OnDERMAND Dermatology, New York,
New York, USA

ANTONELLA TOSTI, MD
Dr. Phillip Frost Department of Dermatology
and Cutaneous Surgery, University of Miami
Miller School of Medicine, Miami, Florida,
USA

CAIWEI ZHENG, BA
University of Miami Miller School of Medicine,
Miami, Florida, USA

Contents

> A number of pathways and factors including oxidative stress, inflammation, prosta-glandins, vasculogenesis, Wnt/β-catenin, and transforming growth factor-β have been shown to be important in male androgenetic alopecia. There is limited but increasing evidence of the potential usefulness of antioxidants, anti-inflammatory agents, prostaglandins, and growth factors for treating of androgenetic alopecia. Lifestyle factors and comorbidities including cardiovascular risk factors have been shown to be associated with male androgenetic alopecia. Further study of these pathways, factors, and comorbidities is needed to better understand the pathophys-iology, find potentially useful therapeutic targets, and ensure a comprehensive approach to the management of androgenetic alopecia in men.

> Hair loss affects millions of people worldwide and can have devastating effects on an individual's psychoemotional well-being. Today hair restoration technologies through hair transplantation have advanced with the use of robots and follicular unit extraction and grafting that it is possible to offer to patient's excellent clinical re-sults. Adjuvant modalities such as platelet-rich plasma injections, lasers, and stem cells can further enhance the durability, health, and appearance of hair transplants.

> The precise and reliable diagnosis of hair loss disorders is essential for developing a successful management plan. It is, thus, the responsibility of the dermatologist to select the appropriate diagnostic tools to effectively evaluate patients presenting with hair loss concerns. Fortunately, there is a growing body of noninvasive and invasive diagnostic resources, each with advantages and disadvantages. For the practicing dermatologist, tactile assessments and direct visualization are enhanced with scoring instruments, questionnaires, handheld trichoscopy, and scalp biopsy. For research and clinical study purposes, the more precise, high-resolution tools such as videodermoscopy, optical coherence tomography, and phototrichograms, may be useful.

> This article focuses on the assessment and treatment of patients with primary cicatricial alopecia and provides new information regarding the genetics and pathophysiology of this group of diseases.

Central centrifugal cicatricial alopecia (CCCA) is the most common form of primary scarring alopecia diagnosed in women of African descent. Although the etiology was originally attributed exclusively to hairstyling practices common among women of African descent, more recent research on CCCA supports the concept that there are several contributing factors, including variants in gene expression, hair grooming practices that increase fragility on the hair follicle, and associations with other systemic conditions. Treatment of CCCA involves a combination of patient counseling and education on alternative hairstyles, medical therapies, and procedural methods when necessary.

Alopecia areata (AA) is a chronic, relapsing, autoimmune disorder characterized by patchy nonscaring hair loss. Although the pathogenesis of alopecia areata is not yet completely elucidated, loss of immune privilege in anagen stage hair follicles is widely accepted to play a key role. Several cytokines that depend on Janus kinase signaling have been identified to be involved in AA, including interleukin (IL)-2, IL-7, IL-15, IL-21, and interferon-γ, making Janus kinase inhibitors an attractive therapeutic target. Available information indicates that about 70% of patients with AA experience significant regrowth, but interruption of treatment is associated with disease recurrence.

Hair loss has a multifactorial etiology that includes internal and external triggers. These include poor diet and nutrition (extrinsic), as well as the natural aging process (intrinsic). Other external factors include pollution, hair products, hair styling, and ultraviolet exposure, which can cause free radical formation, oxidative stress, and microinflammation at the site of the hair follicles. Botanic substances have demonstrated antioxidant, anti-inflammatory, and immune-enhancing properties. Vitamins and minerals are needed when deficiencies are apparent or demonstrate efficacy at higher doses than normally found in one's diet. The safety and efficacy of oral nutraceuticals have been demonstrated in clinical trials.

Current medicinal therapies for treating hair loss have shortcomes due to variability and ineffectiveness, noncompliance, and adverse effects. The prevalence of hair loss and its associated negative psychological impact have driven research into regenerative medicine approaches, such as platelet-rich plasma (PRP) and cell-based therapies, in an attempt to find alternative, safe, effective, and reproducible treatments. Current research shows promising results from these therapies; however, more robust trials are needed to confirm the reported efficacies of PRP and cell-based therapies. Moreover, standardization of treatment preparation as well as dose and regimen are needed.

Limitations to traditional therapies for hair and scalp disorders have spurred significant interest in energy-based devices. Energy-based devices stand apart from traditional hair loss therapies in their proposed mechanism of action and many studies show positive results with device monotherapy. Some preliminary studies have also reported an additive effect on hair growth when combining novel energy-based device treatment and traditional topical therapy. This article covers the use of photobiomodulation (PBM), microneedling, laser therapy (including laser-assisted drug delivery [LADD]), and radiofrequency (RF) in the treatment of hair loss.

This article introduces the reader to the key components of hair transplantation, including evaluating the surgical patient, deciding whether to perform follicular unit transplantation (FUT) or follicular unit extraction (FUE), understanding the key components of these procedures, and establishing practical preoperative and postoperative protocols.

Significant androgenetic hair loss occurs in men older than 50 years, and in women it occurs in many who are perimenopausal, menopausal, and postmenopausal. By age 60 years, it is estimated that 80% of women experience hair loss. Other nonandrogenetic forms of hair loss occur due to various dermatologic disorders as well as systemic disorders. Children may also experience significant hair loss, often due to genetic abnormalities and incidences of trauma. In this article the author discusses a combination approach to hair loss for men, women, and children.

DERMATOLOGIC CLINICS

SERIES OF RELATED INTEREST

Medical Clinics
https://www.medical.theclinics.com/
Primary Care: Clinics in Office Practice
https://www.primarycare.theclinics.com/

THE CLINICS ARE AVAILABLE ONLINE!
Access your subscription at:
www.theclinics.com

Preface
The Hair Comeback

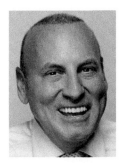

Neil S. Sadick, MD, FACP, FAACS, FACPh, FAAD
Editor

Once a condition thought to happen to men only, hair loss is now widely recognized that it affects people of all ages, genders, and ethnicities with no exceptions. Compared with other dermatologic problems, losing hair carries a lot larger emotional overtone in affected individuals. In this age of innovation, however, with a deep understanding of the causes of hair loss together with advances in diagnostic tools, and a tech revolution in energy-based devices for hair growth and automated hair transplantation, the reversal of hair loss can be a reality. Simply put, the hair comes back.

This special issue of *Dermatologic Clinics* serves as a comprehensive overview of the types and causes of hair loss, the way hair loss is diagnosed, and all the new strategies to treat it. Platelet-rich plasma therapy, the use of fractional lasers and low-level laser therapy, and new-generation nutraceuticals designed for hair are all described in depth in the supplement.

Our aim is to guide dermatologists and dermatologic surgeons, from novices to experienced, to the latest ins and outs of treating hair loss and help them evolve from simply prescribing the one of 2 Food and Drug Administration–approved drugs for hair loss, to a more holistic approach that takes into account the pathophysiology that drives hair loss.

The contributors to the special issue are all outstanding colleagues and experts in their field of research. The editors wish to thank them for their excellent work and for providing updated information and increasing the value of the issue. We hope that this issue covers the wide spectrum of general and specialized hair health care and will provide a thorough account of our present knowledge.

Our hope is that this supplement brings the hair loss patient to the forefront of clinical research and care, so physicians can be intimately attuned to their needs and apply the best treatment strategies to them.

Neil S. Sadick, MD, FACP, FAACS, FACPh, FAAD
Department of Dermatology
Weill Medical College of
Cornell University
New York, NY 10065, USA

Sadick Dermatology
911 Park Avenue, Suite 1A
New York, NY 10075, USA

E-mail address:
nssderm@sadickdermatology.com

Dermatol Clin 39 (2021) ix
https://doi.org/10.1016/j.det.2021.04.005
0733-8635/21/© 2021 Published by Elsevier Inc.

Clinical Patterns of Hair Loss in Men
Is Dihydrotestosterone the Only Culprit?

Natalie Kash, MD[a], Matt Leavitt, DO[a,b,c,d,*], Adam Leavitt, MD[e,1], Spencer D. Hawkins, MD[e,1], Rahil B. Roopani, MD[f]

KEYWORDS

- Alopecia • Androgenetic alopecia • Pathway • Oxidative stress • Inflammation • Prostaglandin • Comorbidities • Risk factors

KEY POINTS

- Pathways and factors, including oxidative stress, inflammation, prostaglandins, vasculogenesis, Wnt/β-catenin, and transforming growth factor-β, have increasingly been shown to be important in the pathophysiology of androgenetic alopecia in men.
- There is limited but increasing evidence of the potential safety and efficacy of treatments targeting these pathways for androgenetic alopecia.
- Lifestyle factors and comorbidities including cardiovascular risk factors have been shown to be associated with male androgenetic alopecia.
- Changes in hair characteristics related to aging, termed senescent alopecia, often coexist with male androgenetic alopecia with advancing age.
- Further study of these pathways, risk factors, and comorbidities is important to better understand the pathophysiology, find potentially useful therapeutic targets, and ensure a comprehensive approach to the management of androgenetic alopecia in men.

INTRODUCTION

The pathophysiology of male androgenetic alopecia (AGA) has focused on the role of androgens, mainly dihydrotestosterone (DHT) and its production by 5α-reductase. Inhibitors of 5α-reductase have been developed and studied for male AGA including finasteride, which was approved by the US Food and Drug Administration for the treatment of male AGA in 1998. Overall, the important role of DHT in the pathophysiology of male AGA and as a therapeutic target has been well-established. However, there is increasing evidence of other important pathways and factors in the development and pathophysiology of male AGA, which are discussed herein.

OXIDATIVE STRESS

Reactive oxygen species (ROS) are created during normal cellular function and have important physiologic functions, including maintenance of β-catenin

Content from this article must be reproduced verbatim, in its entirety, with no modifications. Reprints may not be altered in any way. Please request permissions from Dr. Matt Leavitt at DrMattL@leavittmgt.com.

[a] Department of Dermatology, Kansas City University-Graduate Medical Education Consortium/Advanced Dermatology and Cosmetic Surgery Orlando Dermatology Program, 260 Lookout Place, Suite 103, Maitland, FL 32751, USA; [b] Advanced Dermatology and Cosmetic Surgery, Maitland, FL, USA; [c] University of Central Florida, College of Medicine, Orlando, FL, USA; [d] Bosley Medical Group, Maitland, FL, USA; [e] Department of Dermatology, The University of Michigan, Ann Arbor, MI, USA; [f] Hair Restoration Surgery Program, Leavitt Medical Associates, 260 Lookout Place, Suite 103, Maitland, FL 32751, USA
[1] Present address: 1500 East Medical Center Drive, Ann Arbor, MI 48103, USA.
* Corresponding author. 260 Lookout Place, Suite 103, Maitland, FL 32751.
E-mail address: DrMattL@leavittmgt.com

derm.theclinics.com

and notch signaling during normal hair follicle development and in the cycling of fully developed hair follicles from anagen to catagen.[1–4] Oxidative stress occurs when there is an imbalance between ROS production and normal methods of reduction such as antioxidant function to avoid damage to cell membranes, lipids, protein, and DNA.[4] Lipid peroxidation in particular has been shown to lead to the induction of apoptosis and early catagen in murine hair follicles.[5]

In vitro human studies of men with AGA have shown increased markers of and increased sensitivity to oxidative stress in dermal papilla cells from a balding scalp compared with those from a nonbalding scalp.[6,7] A study analyzing microarray gene expression data from balding and nonbalding scalps in 5 male patients with AGA found upregulated genes in the oxidative stress pathway.[8] In cultured human hair follicles, oxidative stress has been shown to lead to apoptosis and matrix growth inhibition.[9] Activation of the transcription factor, nuclear factor erythroid 2-related factor 2, has been shown to prevent this growth inhibition following ROS exposure, and nuclear factor erythroid 2-related factor 2 activators, including metformin and sulforaphane, have been suggested as potential therapies.[9–11] However, studies of their effect on hair growth have been limited to murine studies, and there is evidence that these agents additionally act on hair growth through other pathways.[10,11]

A number of small case control studies compared serum markers of oxidative stress, including oxidant levels, antioxidant levels, and oxidative stress index. Although the individual methods of measuring oxidative stress differed between studies, generally there were indicators of higher serum oxidative stress in patients with AGA, including early-onset AGA in some studies, compared with age-matched controls.[12–14] Of note, limitations of these studies include small size, lack of prospective data, and measure of serum not follicular oxidative stress. Larger and prospective studies are still needed to better characterize the association and determine the clinical significance and causal or temporal relationship between oxidative stress and AGA.

The demonstration of the importance of oxidative stress in AGA has led to the investigation of a number of antioxidants for the treatment of AGA. There have been limited in vivo human studies on the efficacy of systemic antioxidants; these include a case series on systemic dexpanthenol, a few nonrandomized prospective studies on topical antioxidants, topical melatonin, and oral nutritional supplements, as well as randomized controlled trials on oral tocotrienols, topical procyanidin B-2, topical melatonin, topical herbal extracts, and oral nutritional supplements.[15–28] However, these studies are relatively small with short follow-up periods, some were performed in mostly females, and many include combination therapies with multiple antioxidant, anti-inflammatory, and antiandrogenic agents. Further investigation into their safety and efficacy for male AGA, ideal methods of delivery, dosing, combinations, and larger prospective studies including further comparative studies are still needed.

Additionally, a number of largely speculative studies have proposed that UV exposure may be linked to AGA through direct damage of hair follicles by way of the generation of oxidative stress and a proinflammatory state.[4,29,30] More recently, an in vitro study by Lu and colleagues[31] characterized the response of human hair follicles to UV exposure and found evidence to support oxidative stress, inflammation, and reduced proliferation of hair follicles following UV exposure. Of note, the in vivo clinical significance of UV exposure in AGA has not been studied. Other sources of oxidative stress include inflammation, smoking, poor nutrition, and aging (see corresponding sections elsewhere in this article).[4,30–33]

Further study of the role of oxidative stress and antioxidants in AGA is required to both better understand the pathophysiology of AGA and to determine the potential usefulness of various antioxidants in the treatment of AGA.

INFLAMMATION

The role of inflammation in AGA has been investigated by a number of small studies that performed direct immunofluorescence and histopathologic studies on scalp biopsies from patients with AGA. These studies have reported clear evidence of inflammation including granular deposits of immunoglobulin M or complement component 3 at the basement membrane, activated T-cell infiltrates at the follicular infundibula and follicular bulge, mast cell degranulation and fibroblastic activation in the fibrous sheath, and ultimately fibrosis.[34–38] This inflammation has been termed follicular microinflammation because the process involves a slow, subtle, and indolent course, in contrast with the more robust inflammatory and destructive process in inflammatory scarring alopecias.[29,39]

The precise pathophysiology of this microinflammatory process has yet to be established; however, biopsies from areas of clinically uninvolved scalp in patients with AGA already demonstrate the presence of inflammatory infiltrates and fibrosis, indicating that follicular microinflammation is not a secondary phenomenon but an active participant in pathogenesis.[36,37,40,41] Additionally, there is a correlation between inflammatory infiltrates and apoptosis in miniaturized follicles, suggesting that inflammation can play a role in the pathogenesis of follicle miniaturization.[42] Proinflammatory cytokines like interleukin-1 and tumor necrosis factor-α are also known to induce premature catagen, liberate ROS, cause apoptosis, and further propagate inflammation.[29,43] Transforming growth factor-β may also be implicated because it plays a role in perifollicular fibrosis and miniaturization.[44] Alterations in cytokine and protein expression might not be immediately destructive, but over time they may chronically dysregulate physiologic cycling dynamics and follicle stem cell homeostasis.[29,36,37,41,45,46]

Additionally, more recent studies have found that the extent of inflammation correlates with the most severe clinical forms of AGA, and the addition of anti-inflammatory therapies to AGA treatment has led to improved treatment outcomes.[37,38] Clearly the presence and role of inflammation cannot be ignored in the pathophysiology of hair loss, and future therapeutic approaches to AGA should comprehensively address the multiple factors that affect the follicle including inflammation.[46]

PROSTAGLANDINS

Prostaglandins (PGs) have been actively studied in AGA given their role in inflammation, vasculogenesis, and wound healing.[47] Their generation starts with the release of arachidonic acid from cell membrane phospholipids by phospholipase A_2.[48,49] Arachidonic acid is then metabolized by either PG H synthases (PGHS) or lipoxygenases to form PGH_2 or leukotrienes, respectively.[50] PGH_2 is the precursor of PGD_2, PGE_2, $PGF_{2\alpha}$, prostacyclin (PGI_2), and thromboxane A_2.[51]

Although the exact role of prostanoids in the regulation of hair growth and cycling is unknown, it is clear that there exists a complex homeostasis at the follicular level of products of the arachidonic acid pathway. PGHS enzymes are expressed in hair follicles and sebaceous glands.[52–54] This expression includes the widely distributed PGHS-1 and inducible PGHS-2 isoforms, which have been immunolocalized to the dermal papilla during anagen and catagen.[55] Murine studies have shown evidence of PGD_2 inhibiting hair growth, and a human study in men with AGA found higher protein and messenger RNA levels of PGD_2 synthase enzyme and PGD_2 in bald scalp compared with nonbald scalp.[56,57] Studies in cultured dermal papilla cells have demonstrated that minoxidil stimulates PGE_2 and leukotriene B_4 production and inhibits PGI_2 synthesis.[58]

Perhaps the strongest evidence of the role of PGs on hair cycling has been the serendipitous discovery that topical synthetic $PGF_{2\alpha}$ analogues, including latanoprost and bimatoprost used in the treatment of glaucoma, cause eyelash hypertrichosis.[59] Human clinical trials have found topical bimatoprost, in multiple concentrations and dose frequencies, to be inferior to minoxidil but superior to placebo.[59]

VASCULOGENESIS

The dermal papilla, which controls hair growth, is characterized in the anagen phase by a highly developed vascular network and in the telogen phase by a disappearance of blood vessels in the dermal papilla and the hair bulb.[60] Two studies have investigated the effects of minoxidil on the balding scalp in regards to skin blood flow using laser Doppler velocimetry, with 1 study finding evidence of increased blood flow after the application of a 5% solution and a second failing to find any change in blood flow after the application of a 3% solution.[61,62] Although the effects of topical minoxidil on skin blood flow are nonconclusive, the concept of increased vasculogenesis and its role in hair growth and hair cycling has sparked further research interest.

Vascular endothelial growth factor (VEGF) has a pivotal role in promoting angiogenesis as well as influencing a vast array of cell functions, such as promoting cell survival, proliferation, and generation of nitric oxide and PGI_2.[63] Capillary proliferation during anagen phase has been demonstrated to be temporally and spatially associated with expression of VEGF in the outer root sheath of murine follicles.[64] Additionally, in cultured human dermal papilla cells, minoxidil has been shown to increase VEGF expression in a dose-dependent manner.[60]

Platelet-rich plasma is gaining steam as a new strategy for the treatment of AGA. Although limited by great variation in the methods of its preparation and administration, there is increasing evidence of its efficacy in the treatment of AGA.[65] Additionally, platelet-rich plasma has been shown to contain and lead to increased endogenous expression of a number of growth factors, including VEGF, platelet-derived growth factors, insulin-like growth factor, and epidermal growth factors, which promote angiogenesis and differentiation of cells in the scalp microenvironement.[65]

It is clear that there exists a temporal and spatial relationship between the capillary follicular network and the cycling of hair follicles. Perhaps VEGF plays a central role in this pathway, and minoxidil and platelet-rich plasma may increase VEGF and other growth factors, thereby helping to promote follicular angiogenesis. However, further study is still needed.

WNT/β-CATENIN AND TRANSFORMING GROWTH FACTOR-β PATHWAYS

Decreased Wnt/β-catenin and increased transforming growth factor-β pathway signaling are known to be important in the development of miniaturization and decreased hair growth in AGA through both DHT-dependent and DHT-independent pathways, and recently crosstalk between the Wnt and transforming growth factor-β pathways has been demonstrated in follicles from balding scalp in males with AGA.[8,44,66–69] DHT has been shown to decrease Wnt activity through the upregulation of the Wnt inhibitor, dickkopf-1 (DKK-1).[66] This DKK-1 activity has been shown in in vitro studies to be key to the inhibition of outer root sheath keratinocytic growth by DHT; the inhibition was reversed with neutralizing antibodies to DKK-1.[66] Additionally, balding scalp has been shown to have higher levels of DKK-1 compared with nonbald scalp in patients with AGA.[66] L-Ascorbic acid 2-phosphatase and L-threonate have been shown to repress DHT-induced DKK-1 protein expression in human dermal papilla cells, and L-threonate led to reversal of growth inhibition of outer root sheath cells by DHT.[70,71] These agents show potential in the treatment of AGA although no in vivo studies have been performed.[70,71]

AGING

The scalp is subject to both intrinsic and extrinsic aging, including increased oxidative stress.[4,32,72–75] Intrinsic factors are related to genetic and epigenetic mechanisms, whereas extrinsic factors include ultraviolet radiation, pollution, and chemical treatments, among others.[76] Natural aging is characterized by weathering of the hair shaft, decrease in melanin and hair production, and the development of increasingly dry, thin, dull, and brittle hair.[77] Although many people assume that AGA is associated with aging, some people may never develop it no matter how long they live.[78] Senescent alopecia refers to diffuse scalp hair thinning seen with advanced age in individuals without a family history of hair loss or evidence of pattern balding.

Senescent alopecia was described as a distinct process in the 1980s and is characterized histologically by a modest reduction in the size of otherwise normal hair follicles.[79] This process was contrasted with the miniaturization, inflammation, and fibrosis seen with histologic evaluation of male pattern baldness.[79] However, there has been controversy regarding the existence of senescent alopecia as a distinct clinical entity; some studies suggest that many cases of alopecia in older individuals are AGA and that aging itself is not a cause of hair loss.[80] And although it is true that natural aging does not contribute to a significant loss in the number of hairs, most now accept that the main features of senescent alopecia are decrease in hair diameter and length.[81,82] Additionally, there is now evidence of differential gene expression in senescent alopecia and AGA.[83] Senescent alopecia can also be present concurrently with other types of alopecia, including AGA. In older individuals, this overlap can be quite common.[78,84]

Although much of the dermatology literature on age-associated hair changes focuses on hair loss, it is also important to consider that the diameter, length, curvature, and other structural properties of the hair fibers can impact the overall cosmetic appearance of hair.[39] To limit the effects of natural aging on hair health and combat senescent alopecia, it is important to take a holistic approach. Extrinsic components of natural hair aging can be treated with topical antiaging compounds, including photoprotectors and antioxidants, with varying levels of success.[76] Intrinsic components can also be addressed. When concomitant medical hair loss conditions are present such as AGA, seborrheic dermatitis, or psoriasis, they should be treated accordingly with appropriate medical therapy.[39] It is also important to manage age-related general health problems that can affect the condition of the hair: nutritional, endocrine, psychological, drug-related, substance abuse (including smoking), and multimorbidity (see the Lifestyle and Comorbidities section elsewhere in this article).[39]

LIFESTYLE FACTORS AND COMORBIDITIES

Smoking is hypothesized to contribute to hair loss through reduced blood flow to the follicle, DNA damage, pro-oxidant and proinflammatory effects, effects on collagen and elastin, effects on the protease/antiprotease system, inhibition of aromatase, and increased hydroxylation of estradiol.[4,85] Additionally, nuclear factor erythroid 2-related factor 2 may provide a link between smoking and oxidative stress and be a potential therapeutic target based on studies in other cell types, although further study in hair is still needed.[86,87]

A number of observational cross-sectional studies, case-control studies, and a single study of identical twins have shown a potential association between either smoking, alcohol consumption, diet, working hours, and/or stress and AGA.[85,88–97] Importantly, this research provides an opportunity to counsel AGA patients who smoke on the importance of smoking cessation given the potential connection to AGA in addition to the other numerous well-established negative health outcomes. However, other cross-sectional and case-control studies of male patients with AGA have shown no association between either smoking, alcohol consumption, diet, sleeping habits, and/or work and the incidence of AGA.[91,95,96,98,99]

The link between AGA, including early-onset AGA, in men and cardiovascular disease risk factors has been studied over the last 48 years.[100] Numerous case-control studies, cross-sectional studies, meta-analyses, and 1 prospective cohort study among different populations have investigated the association between AGA and various cardiovascular risk factors, including coronary artery disease, metabolic syndrome, insulin resistance, type II diabetes mellitus, an unfavorable lipid profile, systolic or diastolic hypertension, arteriolosclerosis, and increased body mass index or obesity.[101–112] The majority of studies have concluded that there was an association between male AGA and at least 1 of these cardiovascular risk factors; however, which risk factors have been shown to have a significant association with AGA have varied among different studies. Conversely, a few case-control studies have not found a statistically significant association between AGA and any of the risk factors they evaluated.[113,114] Further, a number of studies not only found an association between AGA and at least 1 risk factor, but also found a correlation between the severity of early-onset male AGA and the degree of cardiovascular risk with largely greater than grade III on the Norwood–Hamilton scale and vertex balding associated with higher risk.[101,104,106–108] Both AGA, especially early-onset AGA, and many cardiovascular risk factors, including metabolic syndrome, insulin resistance, coronary artery disease, and obesity, have been linked to oxidative stress, and a better understanding of oxidative stress and AGA may help to explain its association with other conditions. Additionally, in family clusters of women with polycystic ovarian syndrome, evidence shows that men are also affected with the disease—phenotypically expressed as early-onset AGA.[115–117] In fact, a number of clinical and biochemical profile abnormalities, including insulin resistance, low sex hormone–binding globulin, low follicle-stimulating hormone, and high luteinizing hormone, have been noted to be similar between early-onset male AGA and female polycystic ovarian syndrome, suggesting a possible link and providing a potential mechanism for the association between male AGA and cardiovascular disease risk.[115–119]

Variations in the results of studies investigating associations between AGA and numerous lifestyle factors and comorbidities may reflect differences among different populations studied. Additionally, limitations based on study design include the potential for confounding factors. Clearly, further large well-designed studies adjusting for confounding factors and prospective studies are needed to further try to elucidate what factors are not only associated but potentially causative of alopecia. Additionally, further study into the pathophysiology of potential causative factors are needed to better understand their role in the development of AGA.

SUMMARY

The role of 5α-reductase activity and DHT and its usefulness as a therapeutic target for male AGA has been well-established. Additionally, a number of other contributing factors and pathways have been investigated and shown to be involved in AGA in men. Further studies of these pathways in how they relate to AGA and how these translate to potential therapeutic options are still needed.

CLINICS CARE POINTS

- A number of pathways and factors including oxidative stress, inflammation, prostaglandins, vasculogenesis, Wnt/β-catenin, and transforming growth factor-β have increasingly been shown to be important in the pathophysiology of AGA in men.

- There is limited but increasing evidence of the potential safety and efficacy of treatments targeting these pathways including antioxidants, anti-inflammatory agents, prostaglandins, growth factors promoting vasculogenesis, and promoters of the Wnt/β-catenin pathway for AGA.

- Lifestyle factors and comorbidities including cardiovascular risk factors have been shown to be associated with male AGA.

- Changes in hair characteristics related to aging, termed senescent alopecia, often coexists with male AGA with advancing age.

- Further study of these pathways, risk factors, and comorbidities is important to better understand the pathophysiology, find potentially useful therapeutic targets, and ensure a comprehensive approach to the management of AGA in men.

DISCLOSURE

The authors have nothing to disclose.

REFERENCES

1. Hamanaka RB, Glasauer A, Hoover P, et al. Mitochondrial reactive oxygen species promote epidermal differentiation and hair follicle development. Sci Signal 2013;6(261):ra8.
2. Kloepper JE, Baris OR, Reuter K, et al. Mitochondrial function in murine skin epithelium is crucial for hair follicle morphogenesis and epithelial-mesenchymal interactions. J Invest Dermatol 2015;135(3):679–89.
3. Zhao J, Li H, Zhou R, et al. Foxp1 regulates the proliferation of hair follicle stem cells in response to oxidative stress during hair cycling. PLoS One 2015;10(7):e0131674.
4. Trueb RM. The impact of oxidative stress on hair. Int J Cosmet Sci 2015;37(Suppl 2):25–30.
5. Naito A, Midorikawa T, Yoshino T, et al. Lipid peroxides induce early onset of catagen phase in murine hair cycles. Int J Mol Med 2008;22(6):725–9.
6. Upton JH, Hannen RF, Bahta AW, et al. Oxidative stress-associated senescence in dermal papilla cells of men with androgenetic alopecia. J Invest Dermatol 2015;135(5):1244–52.
7. Bahta AW, Farjo N, Farjo B, et al. Premature senescence of balding dermal papilla cells in vitro is associated with p16(INK4a) expression. J Invest Dermatol 2008;128(5):1088–94.
8. Premanand A, Rajkumari BR. In silico analysis of gene expression data from bald frontal and haired occipital scalp to identify candidate genes in male androgenetic alopecia. Arch Dermatol Res 2019; 311(10):815–24.
9. Haslam IS, Jadkauskaite L, Szabo IL, et al. Oxidative damage control in a human (mini-) organ: Nrf2 activation protects against oxidative stress-induced hair growth inhibition. J Invest Dermatol 2017;137(2):295–304.
10. Chai M, Jiang M, Vergnes L, et al. Stimulation of hair growth by small molecules that activate autophagy. Cell Rep 2019;27(12):3413–21.e3.
11. Sasaki M, Shinozaki S, Shimokado K. Sulforaphane promotes murine hair growth by accelerating the degradation of dihydrotestosterone. Biochem Biophys Res Commun 2016;472(1):250–4.
12. Prie BE, Iosif L, Tivig I, et al. Oxidative stress in androgenetic alopecia. J Med Life 2016;9(1): 79–83.
13. Kaya Erdogan H, Bulur I, Kocaturk E, et al. The role of oxidative stress in early-onset androgenetic alopecia. J Cosmet Dermatol 2017;16(4):527–30.
14. Naziroglu M, Kokcam I. Antioxidants and lipid peroxidation status in the blood of patients with alopecia. Cell Biochem Funct 2000;18(3):169–73.
15. Kutlu O. Dexpanthenol may be a novel treatment for male androgenetic alopecia: analysis of nine cases. Dermatol Ther 2020;33(3):e13381.
16. Anzai A, Pereira AF, Malaquias KR, et al. Efficacy and safety of a new formulation kit (shampoo + lotion) containing anti-inflammatory and antioxidant agents to treat hair loss. Dermatol Ther 2020;33(3): e13293.
17. Beoy LA, Woei WJ, Hay YK. Effects of tocotrienol supplementation on hair growth in human volunteers. Trop Life Sci Res 2010;21(2):91–9.
18. Tenore GC, Caruso D, Buonomo G, et al. Annurca apple nutraceutical formulation enhances keratin expression in a human model of skin and promotes hair growth and tropism in a randomized clinical trial. J Med Food 2018;21(1):90–103.
19. Hatem S, Nasr M, Moftah NH, et al. Clinical cosmeceutical repurposing of melatonin in androgenic alopecia using nanostructured lipid carriers prepared with antioxidant oils. Expert Opin Drug Deliv 2018;15(10):927–35.
20. Hatem S, Nasr M, Moftah NH, et al. Melatonin vitamin C-based nanovesicles for treatment of androgenic alopecia: design, characterization and clinical appraisal. Eur J Pharm Sci 2018;122:246–53.
21. Pekmezci E, Dundar C, Turkoglu M. A proprietary herbal extract against hair loss in androgenetic alopecia and telogen effluvium: a placebo-controlled, single-blind, clinical-instrumental study. Acta Dermatovenerol Alp Pannonica Adriat 2018; 27(2):51–7.
22. Ablon G, Kogan S. A six-month, randomized, double-blind, placebo-controlled study evaluating the safety and efficacy of a nutraceutical supplement for promoting hair growth in women with self-perceived thinning hair. J Drugs Dermatol 2018;17(5):558–65.
23. Nichols AJ, Hughes OB, Canazza A, et al. An open-label evaluator blinded study of the efficacy and safety of a new nutritional supplement in androgenetic alopecia: a pilot study. J Clin Aesthet Dermatol 2017;10(2):52–6.
24. Le Floc'h C, Cheniti A, Connetable S, et al. Effect of a nutritional supplement on hair loss in women. J Cosmet Dermatol 2015;14(1):76–82.
25. Fischer TW, Trueb RM, Hanggi G, et al. Topical melatonin for treatment of androgenetic alopecia. Int J Trichology 2012;4(4):236–45.

26. Fischer TW, Burmeister G, Schmidt HW, et al. Melatonin increases anagen hair rate in women with androgenetic alopecia or diffuse alopecia: results of a pilot randomized controlled trial. Br J Dermatol 2004;150(2):341–5.

27. Takahashi T, Kamimura A, Yokoo Y, et al. The first clinical trial of topical application of procyanidin B-2 to investigate its potential as a hair growing agent. Phytother Res 2001;15(4):331–6.

28. Takahashi T, Kamimura A, Kagoura M, et al. Investigation of the topical application of procyanidin oligomers from apples to identify their potential use as a hair-growing agent. J Cosmet Dermatol 2005;4(4):245–9.

29. Mahe YF, Michelet JF, Billoni N, et al. Androgenetic alopecia and microinflammation. Int J Dermatol 2000;39(8):576–84.

30. Trueb RM. Is androgenetic alopecia a photoaggravated dermatosis? Dermatology 2003;207(4): 343–8.

31. Lu Z, Fischer TW, Hasse S, et al. Profiling the response of human hair follicles to ultraviolet radiation. J Invest Dermatol 2009;129(7):1790–804.

32. Trueb RM. Oxidative stress in ageing of hair. Int J Trichology 2009;1(1):6–14.

33. Seo JA, Bae IH, Jang WH, et al. Hydrogen peroxide and monoethanolamine are the key causative ingredients for hair dye-induced dermatitis and hair loss. J Dermatol Sci 2012;66(1):12–9.

34. Young JW, Conte ET, Leavitt ML, et al. Cutaneous immunopathology of androgenetic alopecia. J Am Osteopath Assoc 1991;91(8):765–71.

35. Jaworsky C, Kligman AM, Murphy GF. Characterization of inflammatory infiltrates in male pattern alopecia: implications for pathogenesis. Br J Dermatol 1992;127(3):239–46.

36. Sueki H, Stoudemayer T, Kligman AM, et al. Quantitative and ultrastructural analysis of inflammatory infiltrates in male pattern alopecia. Acta Derm Venereol 1999;79(5):347–50.

37. El-Domyati M, Attia S, Saleh F, et al. Androgenetic alopecia in males: a histopathological and ultrastructural study. J Cosmet Dermatol 2009;8(2): 83–91.

38. Magro CM, Rossi A, Poe J, et al. The role of inflammation and immunity in the pathogenesis of androgenetic alopecia. J Drugs Dermatol 2011;10(12): 1404–11.

39. Trueb RM, Rezende HD, Dias M. A comment on the science of hair aging. Int J Trichology 2018;10(6): 245–54.

40. Breitkopf T, Leung G, Yu M, et al. The basic science of hair biology: what are the causal mechanisms for the disordered hair follicle? Dermatol Clin 2013;31(1):1–19.

41. Deloche C, de Lacharriere O, Misciali C, et al. Histological features of peripilar signs associated with androgenetic alopecia. Arch Dermatol Res 2004; 295(10):422–8.

42. Ramos PM, Brianezi G, Martins AC, et al. Apoptosis in follicles of individuals with female pattern hair loss is associated with perifollicular microinflammation. Int J Cosmet Sci 2016;38(6):651–4.

43. Trueb RM. Molecular mechanisms of androgenetic alopecia. Exp Gerontol 2002;37(8–9):981–90.

44. Inui S, Fukuzato Y, Nakajima T, et al. Identification of androgen-inducible TGF-beta1 derived from dermal papilla cells as a key mediator in androgenetic alopecia. J Investig Dermatol Symp Proc 2003;8(1):69–71.

45. Leiros GJ, Ceruti JM, Castellanos ML, et al. Androgens modify Wnt agonists/antagonists expression balance in dermal papilla cells preventing hair follicle stem cell differentiation in androgenetic alopecia. Mol Cell Endocrinol 2017;439:26–34.

46. Sadick NS, Callender VD, Kircik LH, et al. New insight into the pathophysiology of hair loss trigger a paradigm shift in the treatment approach. J Drugs Dermatol 2017;16(11):s135–40.

47. Nicolaou A. Eicosanoids in skin inflammation. Prostaglandins Leukot Essent Fatty Acids 2013;88(1): 131–8.

48. Pruzanski W, Vadas P. Phospholipase A2–a mediator between proximal and distal effectors of inflammation. Immunol Today 1991;12(5):143–6.

49. Dennis EA. Diversity of group types, regulation, and function of phospholipase A2. J Biol Chem 1994;269(18):13057–60.

50. Maccarrone M, Putti S, Finazzi Agro A. Nitric oxide donors activate the cyclo-oxygenase and peroxidase activities of prostaglandin H synthase. FEBS Lett 1997;410(2–3):470–6.

51. Messenger AG, Rundegren J. Minoxidil: mechanisms of action on hair growth. Br J Dermatol 2004;150(2):186–94.

52. Colombe L, Vindrios A, Michelet JF, et al. Prostaglandin metabolism in human hair follicle. Exp Dermatol 2007;16(9):762–9.

53. Colombe L, Michelet JF, Bernard BA. Prostanoid receptors in anagen human hair follicles. Exp Dermatol 2008;17(1):63–72.

54. Alestas T, Ganceviciene R, Fimmel S, et al. Enzymes involved in the biosynthesis of leukotriene B4 and prostaglandin E2 are active in sebaceous glands. J Mol Med (Berl) 2006;84(1):75–87.

55. Michelet JF, Commo S, Billoni N, et al. Activation of cytoprotective prostaglandin synthase-1 by minoxidil as a possible explanation for its hair growth-stimulating effect. J Invest Dermatol 1997;108(2): 205–9.

56. Garza LA, Liu Y, Yang Z, et al. Prostaglandin D2 inhibits hair growth and is elevated in bald scalp of men with androgenetic alopecia. Sci Transl Med 2012;4(126):126ra134.

57. Nieves A, Garza LA. Does prostaglandin D2 hold the cure to male pattern baldness? Exp Dermatol 2014;23(4):224–7.

58. Lachgar S, Charveron M, Bouhaddioui N, et al. Inhibitory effects of bFGF, VEGF and minoxidil on collagen synthesis by cultured hair dermal papilla cells. Arch Dermatol Res 1996;288(8):469–73.

59. Barron-Hernandez YL, Tosti A. Bimatoprost for the treatment of eyelash, eyebrow and scalp alopecia. Expert Opin Investig Drugs 2017;26(4):515–22.

60. Lachgar S, Charveron M, Gall Y, et al. Minoxidil up-regulates the expression of vascular endothelial growth factor in human hair dermal papilla cells. Br J Dermatol 1998;138(3):407–11.

61. Wester RC, Maibach HI, Guy RH, et al. Minoxidil stimulates cutaneous blood flow in human balding scalps: pharmacodynamics measured by laser Doppler velocimetry and photopulse plethysmography. J Invest Dermatol 1984;82(5):515–7.

62. Bunker CB, Dowd PM. Alterations in scalp blood flow after the epicutaneous application of 3% minoxidil and 0.1% hexyl nicotinate in alopecia. Br J Dermatol 1987;117(5):668–9.

63. Zachary I, Gliki G. Signaling transduction mechanisms mediating biological actions of the vascular endothelial growth factor family. Cardiovasc Res 2001;49(3):568–81.

64. Yano K, Brown LF, Detmar M. Control of hair growth and follicle size by VEGF-mediated angiogenesis. J Clin Invest 2001;107(4):409–17.

65. Giordano S, Romeo M, di Summa P, et al. A meta-analysis on evidence of platelet-rich plasma for androgenetic alopecia. Int J Trichology 2018; 10(1):1–10.

66. Kwack MH, Sung YK, Chung EJ, et al. Dihydrotestosterone-inducible dickkopf 1 from balding dermal papilla cells causes apoptosis in follicular keratinocytes. J Invest Dermatol 2008;128(2):262–9.

67. Lu GQ, Wu ZB, Chu XY, et al. An investigation of crosstalk between Wnt/beta-catenin and transforming growth factor-beta signaling in androgenetic alopecia. Medicine (Baltimore) 2016; 95(30):e4297.

68. Inui S, Fukuzato Y, Nakajima T, et al. Androgen-inducible TGF-beta1 from balding dermal papilla cells inhibits epithelial cell growth: a clue to understand paradoxical effects of androgen on human hair growth. FASEB J 2002;16(14):1967–9.

69. Kitagawa T, Matsuda K, Inui S, et al. Keratinocyte growth inhibition through the modification of Wnt signaling by androgen in balding dermal papilla cells. J Clin Endocrinol Metab 2009;94(4):1288–94.

70. Kwack MH, Kim MK, Kim JC, et al. L-ascorbic acid 2-phosphate represses the dihydrotestosterone-induced dickkopf-1 expression in human balding dermal papilla cells. Exp Dermatol 2010;19(12):1110–2.

71. Kwack MH, Ahn JS, Kim MK, et al. Preventable effect of L-threonate, an ascorbate metabolite, on androgen-driven balding via repression of dihydrotestosterone-induced dickkopf-1 expression in human hair dermal papilla cells. BMB Rep 2010;43(10):688–92.

72. Harman D. Aging: a theory based on free radical and radiation chemistry. J Gerontol 1956;11(3):298–300.

73. Arck PC, Overall R, Spatz K, et al. Towards a "free radical theory of graying": melanocyte apoptosis in the aging human hair follicle is an indicator of oxidative stress induced tissue damage. FASEB J 2006;20(9):1567–9.

74. Kauser S, Westgate GE, Green MR, et al. Human hair follicle and epidermal melanocytes exhibit striking differences in their aging profile which involves catalase. J Invest Dermatol 2011;131(4):979–82.

75. Huang WY, Huang YC, Huang KS, et al. Stress-induced premature senescence of dermal papilla cells compromises hair follicle epithelial-mesenchymal interaction. J Dermatol Sci 2017; 86(2):114–22.

76. Trueb RM. Pharmacologic interventions in aging hair. Clin Interv Aging 2006;1(2):121–9.

77. Goodier M, Hordinsky M. Normal and aging hair biology and structure 'aging and hair'. Curr Probl Dermatol 2015;47:1–9.

78. Fernandez-Flores A, Saeb-Lima M, Cassarino DS. Histopathology of aging of the hair follicle. J Cutan Pathol 2019;46(7):508–19.

79. Kligman AM. The comparative histopathology of male-pattern baldness and senescent baldness. Clin Dermatol 1988;6(4):108–18.

80. Whiting DA. How real is senescent alopecia? A histopathologic approach. Clin Dermatol 2011;29(1):49–53.

81. Sinclair R, Chapman A, Magee J. The lack of significant changes in scalp hair follicle density with advancing age. Br J Dermatol 2005;152(4):646–9.

82. Courtois M, Loussouarn G, Hourseau C, et al. Ageing and hair cycles. Br J Dermatol 1995; 132(1):86–93.

83. Karnik P, Shah S, Dvorkin-Wininger Y, et al. Microarray analysis of androgenetic and senescent alopecia: comparison of gene expression shows two distinct profiles. J Dermatol Sci 2013;72(2):183–6.

84. Mirmirani P. Age-related hair changes in men: mechanisms and management of alopecia and graying. Maturitas 2015;80(1):58–62.

85. Trüeb RM. Association between smoking and hair loss: another opportunity for health education against smoking? Dermatology 2003;206(3):189–91.

86. Jadkauskaite L, Coulombe PA, Schafer M, et al. Oxidative stress management in the hair follicle:

could targeting NRF2 counter age-related hair disorders and beyond? Bioessays 2017;39(8):1–9.

87. Prasad S, Sajja RK, Kaisar MA, et al. Role of Nrf2 and protective effects of Metformin against tobacco smoke-induced cerebrovascular toxicity. Redox Biol 2017;12:58–69.

88. Su LH, Chen TH. Association of androgenetic alopecia with smoking and its prevalence among Asian men: a community-based survey. Arch Dermatol 2007;143(11):1401–6.

89. Mosley JG, Gibbs AC. Premature gray hair and hair loss among smokers: a new opportunity for health education? Br Med J 1996;313:1616.

90. Salem AS, Ibrahim HS, Abdelaziz HH, et al. Implications of cigarette smoking on early-onset androgenetic alopecia: a cross-sectional Study. J Cosmet Dermatol 2021;20(4):1318–24.

91. Yeo IK, Jang WS, Min PK, et al. An epidemiological study of androgenic alopecia in 3114 Korean patients. Clin Exp Dermatol 2014;39(1):25–9.

92. Fortes C, Mastroeni S, Mannooranparampil T, et al. Mediterranean diet: fresh herbs and fresh vegetables decrease the risk of Androgenetic Alopecia in males. Arch Dermatol Res 2018;310(1):71–6.

93. Son KH, Suh BS, Jeong HS, et al. Relationship between working hours and probability to take alopecia medicine among Korean male workers: a 4-year follow-up study. Ann Occup Environ Med 2019;31:e12.

94. Gatherwright J, Liu MT, Amirlak B, et al. The contribution of endogenous and exogenous factors to male alopecia: a study of identical twins. Plast Reconstr Surg 2013;131(5):794e–801e.

95. Severi G, Sinclair R, Hopper JL, et al. Androgenetic alopecia in men aged 40-69 years: prevalence and risk factors. Br J Dermatol 2003;149(6):1207–13.

96. Fortes C, Mastroeni S, Mannooranparampil TJ, et al. The combination of overweight and smoking increases the severity of androgenetic alopecia. Int J Dermatol 2017;56(8):862–7.

97. Lai CH, Chu NF, Chang CW, et al. Androgenic alopecia is associated with less dietary soy, lower [corrected] blood vanadium and rs1160312 1 polymorphism in Taiwanese communities. PLoS One 2013;8(12):e79789.

98. Gupta S, Goyal I, Mahendra A. Quality of life assessment in patients with androgenetic alopecia. Int J Trichology 2019;11(4):147–52.

99. Salman KE, Altunay IK, Kucukunal NA, et al. Frequency, severity and related factors of androgenetic alopecia in dermatology outpatient clinic: hospital-based cross-sectional study in Turkey. An Bras Dermatol 2017;92(1):35–40.

100. Predicting coronary artery disease. Br Med J 1972; 4(5831):3.

101. Trieu N, Eslick GD. Alopecia and its association with coronary heart disease and cardiovascular risk factors: a meta-analysis. Int J Cardiol 2014; 176(3):687–95.

102. Kim MW, Shin IS, Yoon HS, et al. Lipid profile in patients with androgenetic alopecia: a meta-analysis. J Eur Acad Dermatol Venereol 2017;31(6):942–51.

103. Sharma K, Humane D, Shah K, et al. Androgenic alopecia, premature graying, and hair thinning as independent predictors of coronary artery disease in young Asian males. Cardiovasc Endocrinol 2017;6(4):152–8.

104. Triantafyllidi H, Grafakos A, Ikonomidis I, et al. Severity of alopecia predicts coronary changes and arterial stiffness in untreated hypertensive men. J Clin Hypertens (Greenwich) 2017;19(1): 51–7.

105. Banger HS, Malhotra SK, Singh S, et al. Is early onset androgenic alopecia a marker of metabolic syndrome and carotid artery atherosclerosis in young Indian male patients? Int J Trichology 2015;7(4):141–7.

106. Park SY, Oh SS, Lee WS. Relationship between androgenetic alopecia and cardiovascular risk factors according to BASP classification in Koreans. J Dermatol 2016;43(11):1293–300.

107. Sharma KH, Jindal A. Association between androgenetic alopecia and coronary artery disease in young male patients. Int J Trichology 2014;6(1): 5–7.

108. Ertas R, Orscelik O, Kartal D, et al. Androgenetic alopecia as an indicator of metabolic syndrome and cardiovascular risk. Blood Press 2016;25(3): 141–8.

109. Bakry OA, Shoeib MA, El Shafiee MK, et al. Androgenetic alopecia, metabolic syndrome, and insulin resistance: is there any association? A case-control study. Indian Dermatol Online J 2014;5(3):276–81.

110. Vora RV, Kota R, Singhal RR, et al. Clinical profile of androgenic alopecia and its association with cardiovascular risk factors. Indian J Dermatol 2019; 64(1):19–22.

111. Gopinath H, Upadya GM. Metabolic syndrome in androgenic alopecia. Indian J Dermatol Venereol Leprol 2016;82(4):404–8.

112. Swaroop MR, Kumar BM, Sathyanarayana BD, et al. The association of metabolic syndrome and insulin resistance in early-onset androgenetic alopecia in males: a case-control study. Indian J Dermatol 2019;64(1):23–7.

113. Danesh-Shakiba M, Poorolajal J, Alirezaei P. Androgenetic alopecia: relationship to anthropometric indices, blood pressure and life-style habits. Clin Cosmet Investig Dermatol 2020;13:137–43.

114. Abdel Fattah NS, Darwish YW. Androgenetic alopecia and insulin resistance: are they truly associated? Int J Dermatol 2011;50(4):417–22.

115. Di Guardo F, Ciotta L, Monteleone M, et al. Male equivalent polycystic ovarian syndrome: hormonal,

metabolic, and clinical aspects. Int J Fertil Steril 2020;14(2):79–83.

116. Cannarella R, Condorelli RA, Mongioi LM, et al. Does a male polycystic ovarian syndrome equivalent exist? J Endocrinol Invest 2018;41(1):49–57.

117. Sanke S, Chander R, Jain A, et al. A comparison of the hormonal profile of early androgenetic alopecia in men with the phenotypic equivalent of polycystic ovarian syndrome in women. JAMA Dermatol 2016; 152(9):986–91.

118. Cannarella R, Condorelli RA, Dall'Oglio F, et al. Increased DHEAS and decreased total testosterone serum levels in a subset of men with early-onset androgenetic alopecia: does a male PCOS-equivalent exist? Int J Endocrinol 2020;2020: 1942126.

119. Cannarella R, La Vignera S, Condorelli RA, et al. Glycolipid and hormonal profiles in young men with early-onset androgenetic alopecia: a meta-analysis. Sci Rep 2017;7(1):7801.

Understanding Causes of Hair Loss in Women

Neil Sadick, MD[a,b,c],*, Suleima Arruda, MD[a,c]

KEYWORDS

- Inflammation • Androgenetic alopecia • Female pattern hair loss

KEY POINTS

- Selection of hair transplantation methodology depends on patient goals, type of hair loss, and quality of hair.
- Robotic hair transplantation is the latest frontier in hair restoration.
- Platelet-rich plasma, low-level laser therapy, and stem cells can be used together with hair transplantation to enhance graft survival.

INTRODUCTION

Hair loss in women, also known as female pattern hair loss (FPHL), is a common form of nonscarring hair loss that affects around 20% of adult women in the United States. It is characterized by progressive loss of terminal hairs over the frontal and vertex regions of the scalp, resulting in visible hair thinning. FPHL mostly affects White women compared with Asian and black women. FPHL usually starts after the onset of menopause, although it can also affect women of younger ages. A British study of 377 women who presented to a general dermatology clinic with concerns unrelated to hair loss, 38% of women over the age of 70 years had FPHL.[1] Women with FPHL experience negative psychosocial effects such as feelings of negative body image, poorer self-esteem, and a decreased sense of control over their lives.

The diagnosis of FPHL is usually made clinically, based on the patient history, laboratory tests, and physical examination. The diagnosis is suggested by the detection of a decrease in hair density in the characteristic distribution and an increased prevalence of miniaturized hairs. Skin biopsies are not usually performed, but can be helpful when the diagnosis is uncertain or when a concomitant scalp disorder is suspected.

The progressive thinning and decrease of hair in FPHL results from an ongoing decrease in the ratio of terminal hairs to shorter, thinner vellus hairs in the affected areas, a process known as follicular miniaturization. Consequently, the anagen phase of the hair follicles shortens from a normal duration of a few years to only weeks to months. Although androgens and genetic susceptibility in male androgenetic alopecia are well-accepted factors underlying its pathophysiology, the degree to which these factors contribute to FPHL in most women is less clear; thus, the mechanism through which follicular transformation occurs in FPHL is not completely understood. Today, a combination of hormonal dysregulation, environmental stress, and genetics are thought to collectively contribute to the microinflammation that ultimately leads to FPHL.

EFFECT OF HORMONES

The implication of androgens in the pathophysiology of hair loss is thought to be the most

[a] Department of Dermatology, Weill Medical College of Cornell University, 1305 York Ave 9th Floor, New York, NY 10021, USA; [b] Department of Dermatology, University of Minnesota, Minneapolis, MN 55455, USA; [c] Sadick Dermatology, 911 Park Avenue, New York, NY 10075, USA
* Corresponding author. Department of Dermatology, Weill Medical College of Cornell University, 1305 York Ave 9th Floor, New York, NY 10021.
E-mail address: nssderm@sadickdermatology.com

Dermatol Clin 39 (2021) 371–374
https://doi.org/10.1016/j.det.2021.03.002

elucidated of hair loss triggers, yet ongoing research continuously reveals new mechanism of androgen action. Microinflammation and perifollicular fibrosis has been documented by a plethora of peer-reviewed clinical studies of androgenetic alopecia, highlighting that a key consequence of androgens is triggering a cascade of numerous immune and inflammatory processes.[2–6] Androgens present in both men and women influence hair growth by stimulating the dermal papilla cells to overproduce transforming growth factor-β, which is normally produced in these cells to signal catagen and regression and production of transforming growth factor-β by the dermal papilla cells was shown to induce oxidative stress, as well as perifollicular fibrosis and inflammation via the surrounding fibroblasts.[7] New research also shows that androgens also impair dermal papilla-induced hair follicle stem cell differentiation by inhibiting Wnt signaling, a pathway crucial for anagen entry.[8] Even in the absence of excess androgens, such as in men castrated after puberty, engagement of their downstream effectors suffices to results in the dysregulated pathophysiology seen in hair loss.[9] A steep decrease in estrogen in menopausal women can allow androgen dominance, or even the mere loss of estrogen protection can allow manifestation of androgenetic alopecia in women.

ENVIRONMENTAL AND GENETIC TRIGGERS

The hair follicle is a conduit for intensive interactions with the internal and external environment. Although the effects of extrinsic and intrinsic factors are readily recognized in skin photoaging, their influence in hair follicle biology is underappreciated.[10,11] Nevertheless, a study examining the contribution of endogenous and exogenous factors in the development and severity of male pattern hair loss in 92 genetically identical male twins found that several nongenetic exogenous factors not only contributed significantly to hair loss, but that their effects were also expressed in a distinct spatiotemporal fashion.[12] Both extrinsic triggers such as UV, pollutants, tobacco, and pathogens and intrinsic factors such as genetics, aging, and poor nutrition, target and attack the hair follicle generating oxidative stress and mediating inflammation-associated injury. Both these processes play a central role in the pathophysiology of hair disease, in a manner similar to that seen in chronic diseases, including cancer, aging, diabetes, and cardiovascular and chronic kidney disease, by initiating intracellular signaling cascades that enhance proinflammatory gene expression (tumor necrosis factor α, IL-1), and liberating

reactive oxidative species. For example, the effects exerted by UV radiation on hair follicles are known to be in part mediated via the generation of reactive oxidative species, which induces cell apoptosis and cycle arrest. Preclinical studies have shown that antioxidants such as vitamins E and C can provide photoprotection against oxidative damage.[13]

Genetics also play a role in all manifestations of hair loss, and the genetic make-up of an individual can predispose them to various types of hair disorders (androgenetic alopecia, telogen effluvium, alopecia areata [AA]). Although the androgen receptor was a main candidate gene involved in hair loss susceptibility, recent genetic studies have revealed several additional susceptibility genetic loci involving cell proliferation, perturbed neurologic pathways, altered immune response, and WNT signaling as central drivers of the hair loss process.[14–17] These data further highlight that altered function of molecular pathways lie at the root of hair loss physiology, and that targeting the androgen-dependent pathway does not suffice to effectively combat hair loss. Aside from genetic predisposition that cannot be changed, genetic research has recently shown that epigenetic modification through exogenous and endogenous factors can regulate gene expression, opening an opportunity to therapeutically intervene to rebalance a genetic environment susceptible to hair loss.[18] There is substantial evidence, for instance, that plant phytonutrients can alter the internal environment by epigenetically modifying the transcription of anti-inflammatory and antioxidant genes and such function can be exploited for treatment of hair loss.[19]

CHRONIC STRESS (ELEVATED CORTISOL AND OTHER MEDIATORS OF STRESS)

Although psychoemotional stress was anecdotally associated with hair loss, the underlying science driving this phenomenon was only recently recognized and elucidated. Aside from external and internal environmental triggers, given the dense perifollicular meshwork of sensory nerve endings that are closely associated with mast cells, endothelial cells, and macrophages, hair follicles are also a target of immunomodulatory and neuroendocrine stress mediators including substance P, cortisol, and adrenocorticotropic hormone.[20] Upon stress triggers, nerve fibers secrete neuropeptides such as substance P and nerve growth factor with proinflammatory properties that lead to mast cell degranulation and the release of myriad proinflammatory mediators, such as histamine and tumor necrosis factor α, into the interfollicular tissue,[21] and up-regulation of MHC class I and II microglobulin expression, that trigger the collapse of the hair follicle immune privilege.[22–24] Chronically high stress levels also lead to the production of stress hormones, like cortisol, which are known to cause catagen induction. Moreover, aside from the paracrine action of external hormones, the hair follicle can produce its own stress hormones (adrenocorticotropic hormone, corticotropin-releasing hormone, and cortisol) because it has a fully functional equivalent of the classical hypothalamic–pituitary–adrenal axis, with established regulatory feedback loops. In this way, stress exposure can trigger the hair follicle to secrete its own stress hormones that further dysregulate the hair follicle milieu.

DISCUSSION

The pathophysiology of hair loss is unequivocally extremely complex, involving a plethora of signaling pathways from multiple cell types. Data underscore the flaws of designing androgen-targeting therapies for hair loss, because it is clear that the complex dysregulated signaling is what ultimately causes hair loss, and provided the impetus to shift the therapeutic approach from monotargeting to comprehensively multitargeting aberrant signaling pathways.

Regardless of the trigger, however, the cause of hair disorders is a hair follicle that has lost its homeostatic regulation. Both the hair–brain axis and the environment–hair axis can influence the hair follicle, chisel against its regulatory circuitry, and, in the absence of strategies to counterbalance this attack, can ultimately override the hair follicle's internal controls. The result is exerting a permanent alteration in hair follicle function that renders it in a state of imbalance and establishes deleterious self-sustained inflammatory cascades as the new status quo.

Restoring hair follicles to a state of biological balance requires embracing a new outlook in terms of therapeutics. Current pharmacologic interventions focus mainly on targeting local regulatory circuits, such as hair follicle testosterone metabolism and growth factor pathways. Notably the 2 therapeutic agents approved by the US Food and Drug Administration and European Medicines Agency for the treatment of androgenetic alopecia are topical minoxidil and oral finasteride (1 mg/d).[25] However, both these agents have had a limited success rate, and even worse, unfavorable side effects, including sexual dysfunction. More important, these therapies rely on monotargeting specific molecules, rather than considering the underlying pathophysiology of activated of proinflammatory, profibrotic cascades and the presence of microinflammation. Thus, there needs to be a paradigm shift in approaching hair loss treatments, one that targets not only androgens but also inflammation, oxidative stress, elevated stress mediators like cortisol, and their downstream signaling mediators. In addition, the treatment should stimulate a nutrient-rich microenvironment in the hair follicle niche to promote repair and structural regeneration. Therapies such as nutraceuticals, platelet-rich plasma, and low-level laser therapy are slowly but surely emerging and are increasingly recognized for their efficacy either as a standalone treatment regime or combined with traditional hair loss treatments.[26–29] Nutraceuticals contain potent botanicals with antioxidant, anti-inflammatory, and growth-promoting properties that can target multiple triggers underlying hair loss.[30] By targeting multiple triggers at once, as well as optimizing and recalibrating the immune response, these new therapeutic approaches present a more comprehensive solution to restoring the imbalance of the disordered follicle. Autologous platelet-rich plasma injections have been used for almost a decade now in female and male hair loss, and have a documented positive effect in restoring hair loss, most likely owing to the anti-inflammatory action of the preparation. Low-level laser therapy and even energy-based devices such as microneedling radiofrequency or fractional lasers have also shown promise in this multimodal therapeutic approach as the localized microwounds and consequent wound healing processes that are activated in the scalp region, allow recruiting of dermal papilla stem cells, dampening of inflammation and finally follicular growth.

CLINICS CARE POINTS

- Hair loss has a complex etiology stemming from chronic inflammation due to hormones, genetics, stress and other environmental factors.
- Treatment of hair loss in women should be based on a combination approach that considers the underlying pathophysiology.
- New generation approaches such as platelet-rich plasma, energy-based devices, and advanced nutraceuticals can provide optimal clinical results for reduction of hair loss and long-term hair health.

DISCLOSURE

Nothing to disclose.

REFERENCES

1. Hutchinson PE. Hair density, hair diameter and the prevalence of female pattern hair loss. Br J Dermatol 2002;146(5):922–3 [author reply: 923–4].

2. Deloche C, de Lacharriere O, Misciali C, et al. Histological features of peripilar signs associated with androgenetic alopecia. Arch Dermatol Res 2004; 295(10):422–8.

3. El-Domyati M, Attia S, Saleh F, et al. Androgenetic alopecia in males: a histopathological and ultrastructural study. J Cosmet Dermatol 2009;8(2):83–91.

4. Magro CM, Rossi A, Poe J, et al. The role of inflammation and immunity in the pathogenesis of androgenetic alopecia. J Drugs Dermatol 2011;10(12): 1404–11.

5. Nirmal B, Somiah S, Sacchidanand SA, et al. Evaluation of perifollicular inflammation of donor area during hair transplantation in androgenetic alopecia and its comparison with controls. Int J Trichol 2013;5(2):73–6.

6. Ramos PM, Brianezi G, Martins AC, et al. Apoptosis in follicles of individuals with female pattern hair loss is associated with perifollicular microinflammation. Int J Cosmet Sci 2016;38(6):651–4.

7. Shin H, Yoo HG, Inui S, et al. Induction of transforming growth factor-beta 1 by androgen is mediated by reactive oxygen species in hair follicle dermal papilla cells. BMB Rep 2013;46(9):460–4.

8. Leiros GJ, Ceruti JM, Castellanos ML, et al. Androgens modify Wnt agonists/antagonists expression balance in dermal papilla cells preventing hair follicle stem cell differentiation in androgenetic alopecia. Mol Cell Endocrinol 2017;439:26–34.

9. Randall VA. Hormonal regulation of hair follicles exhibits a biological paradox. Semin Cell Dev Biol 2007;18(2):274–85.

10. Lee WS. Photoaggravation of hair aging. Int J Trichol 2009;1(2):94–9.

11. Trueb RM. Is androgenetic alopecia a photoaggravated dermatosis? Dermatology 2003;207(4):343–8.

12. Gatherwright J, Liu MT, Amirlak B, et al. The contribution of endogenous and exogenous factors to male alopecia: a study of identical twins. Plast Reconstr Surg 2013;131(5):794e–801e.

13. Fernandez E, Martinez-Teipel B, Armengol R, et al. Efficacy of antioxidants in human hair. J Photochem Photobiol B 2012;117:146–56.

14. Dey-Rao R, Sinha AA. A genomic approach to susceptibility and pathogenesis leads to identifying potential novel therapeutic targets in androgenetic alopecia. Genomics 2017.

15. Hagenaars SP, Hill WD, Harris SE, et al. Genetic prediction of male pattern baldness. PLoS Genet 2017; 13(2):e1006594.

16. Heilmann-Heimbach S, Herold C, Hochfeld LM, et al. Meta-analysis identifies novel risk loci and yields systematic insights into the biology of male-pattern baldness. Nat Commun 2017;8:14694.

17. Heilmann-Heimbach S, Hochfeld LM, Paus R, et al. Hunting the genes in male-pattern alopecia: how important are they, how close are we and what will they tell us? Exp Dermatol 2016;25(4):251–7.

18. Banka N, Bunagan MJ, Shapiro J. Pattern hair loss in men: diagnosis and medical treatment. Dermatol Clin 2013;31(1):129–40.

19. Huang J, Plass C, Gerhauser C. Cancer chemoprevention by targeting the epigenome. Curr Drug Targets 2011;12(13):1925–56.

20. Paus R, Theoharides TC, Arck PC. Neuroimmunoendocrine circuitry of the 'brain-skin connection'. Trends Immunol 2006;27(1):32–9.

21. Arck PC, Handjiski B, Peters EM, et al. Stress inhibits hair growth in mice by induction of premature catagen development and deleterious perifollicular inflammatory events via neuropeptide substance P-dependent pathways. Am J Pathol 2003;162(3): 803–14.

22. Baluk P. Neurogenic inflammation in skin and airways. J Investig Dermatol Symp Proc 1997;2(1): 76–81.

23. Peters EM, Arck PC, Paus R. Hair growth inhibition by psychoemotional stress: a mouse model for neural mechanisms in hair growth control. Exp Dermatol 2006;15(1):1–13.

24. Peters EM, Liotiri S, Bodo E, et al. Probing the effects of stress mediators on the human hair follicle: substance P holds central position. Am J Pathol 2007;171(6):1872–86.

25. Kelly Y, Blanco A, Tosti A. Androgenetic alopecia: an update of treatment options. Drugs 2016;76(14): 1349–64.

26. Ablon G. A 6-month, randomized, double-blind, placebo-controlled study evaluating the ability of a marine complex supplement to promote hair growth in men with thinning hair. J Cosmet Dermatol 2016; 15(4):358–66.

27. Afifi L, Maranda EL, Zarei M, et al. Low-level laser therapy as a treatment for androgenetic alopecia. Lasers Surg Med 2017;49(1):27–39.

28. Ferneini EM, Beauvais D, Castiglione C, et al. Platelet-rich plasma in androgenic alopecia: indications, technique, and potential benefits. J Oral Maxillofac Surg 2016.

29. Gupta AK, Foley KA. A critical assessment of the evidence for low-level laser therapy in the treatment of hair loss. Dermatol Surg 2017;43(2):188–97.

30. Rinaldi S, Bussa M, Mascaro A. Update on the treatment of androgenetic alopecia. Eur Rev Med Pharmacol Sci 2016;20(1):54–8.

New Diagnostic Tools to Evaluate Hair Loss

Alana Kurtti, BS[a,b], Jared Jagdeo, MD, MS[b,c], Amanda Eisinger, DO[d],
Kumar Sukhdeo, MD, PhD[d,*]

KEYWORDS

• Hair • Imaging • Trichoscopy • Methods • Diagnostics

KEY POINTS

- Early and accurate diagnosis of hair loss disorders is essential for successful management.
- Tactile assessments and direct visualization are enhanced with analog and digital imaging devices, as well as scoring rubrics and histology.
- Research and clinical studies may benefit from precision instrumentation with high resolution.

INTRODUCTION

Concern for hair loss is among the most common encounters in outpatient dermatologic clinics.[1] Treatment plans are predicated on correct diagnoses after obtaining a thorough history and examination, including visual and tactile elements. Intrinsic hair follicle pathophysiology, as with androgen-driven pattern hair loss, is the most common cause of alopecia; however, extrinsic factors within the scalp and manipulation of the hair shaft also need consideration.[2] Misdiagnosis is not uncommon and can lead to disease progression, clinical delay, frustration, expense, and mistrust. Because patients are often keen to halt or reverse hair loss, a diagnosis supplemented with metrics to stage and/or grade disease progression is useful, particularly in follow-up encounters. In this review, we provide an update on the growing diagnostic armamentarium to assist the visual and tactile assessment of hair loss (**Table 1**).

NONINVASIVE METHODS
Questionnaires

A questionnaire is a simple, time-saving method for gathering detailed patient information that may yield more comprehensive patient histories, provide valuable clues for diagnosis, and facilitate monitoring treatment response. Several validated questionnaires exist for assessing behavioral and lifestyle influence on hair loss, patient perception of treatment response, and satisfaction with appearance.[3,4] Dermatologists may also use questionnaires to assess quality of life impact, because hair loss disorders have profound consequences on patient self-esteem and mental health.[5] For example, the hairdex questionnaire is a patient-oriented instrument used for evaluation of quality of life in patients suffering from hair diseases.[6] Because time is often limited for each visit, having the patient complete a questionnaire in advance elicits necessary information, saves time, and makes patients feel heard.

Hair Counts

Daily hair counts facilitate the quantification of patient hair loss and differentiate pathologic hair loss from physiologic shedding. Patients are instructed to collect and count all hairs shed each day for the course of a week.[7] Although historically considered normal for patients to lose up to 100 hairs per day, this number was derived from a

Funding sources: None.
[a] Rutgers Robert Wood Johnson Medical School, Piscataway, NJ 08854, USA; [b] Dermatology Service, VA New York Harbor Healthcare System, Brooklyn, NY 11209, USA; [c] Department of Dermatology, SUNY Downstate Medical Center, Brooklyn, NY 11203, USA; [d] Pilaris, OnDERMAND Dermatology, New York, NY 10022, USA
* Corresponding author. 635 Madison Avenue Suite 1402, New York, NY 10022.
E-mail address: kumar@pilaris.com

Dermatol Clin 39 (2021) 375–381
https://doi.org/10.1016/j.det.2021.03.003
0733-8635/21/© 2021 Elsevier Inc. All rights reserved.

Table 1
Diagnostic test categorized by invasiveness

Noninvasive	Semi-invasive	Invasive
Questionnaires	Hair pull	Biopsy
Hair counts	Modified wash test	
Card test	Hair clipping (microscopy and TrichoScan)	
Grading systems	Optical coherence tomography	
Global photography		
Dermoscopy/ videodermoscopy		
Folliscope		
Raman spectroscopy		

mathematical equation and has not been validated by a clinical study or standardized method.[8,9] Additionally, maintaining daily hair counts is cumbersome and may yield inaccurate results because many shed hairs are not detected.[9] A more reliable and practical method for quantifying hair loss proposed is the 60-second hair count. Using this method, before shampooing, the patient combs their hair for 60 seconds over a pillow or sheet of contrasting color to their hair and counts the number of hairs shed.[9] This is repeated before 3 consecutive shampooings. These counts are performed monthly for a duration of 6 months. Wasko and colleagues[9] sought to define the normal range for the 60-second hair count, revealing the normal shedding range to be 0 to 78 hairs, with a mean of 10.2 hairs in 20- to 40-year-old men and a range of 0 to 43 hairs, with a mean of 10.3 hairs, in 41- to 60-year-old men.

Card Test

The card test is a simple, noninvasive technique that enables the visualization and assessment of distal hair shaft tips. The clinician places a card markedly different in color from the patient's hair color (eg, a white card for black hair) against a section of the scalp to visualize hair strands against the card.[10] The clinician may observe miniaturized hair or new hair growth and differentiate new hair, indicated by tapered tips, from cut or broken hair, indicated by sharp tips.[11] This test is useful for the diagnosis of androgenetic alopecia (AGA) and

telogen effluvium (TE), because miniature hairs can be observed in the androgen-dependent areas of both men and women with AGA and, in a regrowing TE, a short frontal fringe is typically observed.[8]

Grading Systems

Hair shedding scale

Hair shedding scales are fast, effective tools that provide semiquantitative metrics of hair loss activity or treatment response. The Sinclair Hair Shedding Scale consists of 6 paneled images depicting increasing amounts of shedding, with the loss of 100 hair shafts representing normal daily shed. Patients self-assess which image best corresponds with the amount of hair shed on an average day.[12] Hair shedding scales also exist for short, medium, and long hair to account for differences in shaft length, but additional reference standards need development in different curl patterns, such as African hair. Although these simple tools are useful for discriminating normal from excessive shedding in a busy office practice, the hair-shedding scale is not a comprehensive diagnostic instrument.[13]

Hamilton–Norwood scale

The Hamilton–Norwood Scale is the leading classification system used to determine the severity of AGA. The scale is divided into 7 stages and provides a visual representation of the progressive grades of male pattern baldness. However, not all men with AGA follow hair loss patterns depicted by the Hamilton–Norwood Scale. Studies have shown that 10% of men have a pattern that resembles female AGA.[14]

Ludwig scale

The Ludwig scale is the leading classification system used to grade female pattern hair loss (FPHL). The scale is a visual depiction of 3 progressive grades of hair loss, consisting of thinning on the crown with preservation of the frontal hairline. Although popular, the Ludwig scale has several limitations. For one, it fails to detect early-stage FPHL because it focuses on obvious crown thinning and neglects alternative patterns, such as the Christmas tree hair loss pattern in the fronto-vertical area described by Olsen.[15] Additionally, females with male patterned hair loss cannot be classified with this tool.[16]

Female Pattern Hair Loss Severity Index

Harries and colleagues[17] proposed a new tool, the Female Pattern Hair Loss Severity Index (FPHL-SI) for earlier diagnosis and monitoring of FPHL. The FPHL-SI is a 3-component severity scale that combines validated measures of hair shedding, midline hair density, and scalp trichoscopy criteria to produce a total FPHL-SI score (maximum score = 20).[17] A score of 0 to 4 makes FPHL unlikely and 5 to 9 indicates early-stage FPHL, with higher scores indicating greater disease severity.[17] The FPHL-SI is a simple system of sufficient sensitivity to diagnose early FPHL and monitor changes.[17]

Severity of Alopecia Tool Score

The Severity of Alopecia Tool Score is a simple tool used for determining the severity of alopecia. Traditionally, the score was determined with the help of a figure aid by adding the percentage hair loss in each of 4 views of the scalp.[18] In 2016, the figure was updated to include smaller increments of scalp coverage to facilitate the assessment of hair loss where small patches of hair loss predominate, such as in alopecia areata, and where only certain areas of the scalp are involved, such as in MPHL.[19] Although useful, manually estimating percentages for a Severity of Alopecia Tool Score is not easily reproducible because there is great inter-rater variability, even among expert clinicians.[18] To alleviate this issue, a digital imaging program used to produce automated Severity of Alopecia Tool Score scores was recently developed and validated on a dataset of 250 images of more than 100 patients.[20]

Lichen Planopilaris Activity Index

The Lichen Planopilaris Activity Index is used to quantify the signs and symptoms of lichen planopilaris and frontal fibrosing alopecia. With this instrument, the clinician assigns numeric scores to several subjective and objective variables, including symptoms (pruritus, pain, and burning), signs (erythema, perifollicular erythema, and scale), anagen pull test results, and extent of disease.[21] Although the Lichen Planopilaris Activity Index is comprehensive and validated for lichen planopilaris, the tool has met criticism because it relies on several subjective factors and has not been validated for reliability or use in frontal fibrosing alopecia.[22] In 2017, Saceda-Corralo and colleagues[23] developed and validated the Frontal Fibrosing Alopecia Severity Score, a scoring tool based on weighted clinical signs and associated symptoms, and determined it to be a reliable measure of frontal fibrosing alopecia severity.

Imaging

Global photography

The global photographic assessment is valuable for diagnosis, assessing the degree of hair loss and monitoring clinical changes over time in a consistent fashion. Most electronic medical records allow for rapid capture of images, which can be performed by an assistant in advance. Moreover, a second set of photos taken with the patient's camera phone allows for home comparisons. A reproducible method of photography is recommended. For example, with the patient seated, hair parted down the midline, and with eyes closed, take a series of arms-length photographs to include head-on, side profile (left/right), and birds-eye views. For more precise sequential monitoring with consistent angles, magnification, and lighting, a stereotactic positioning device (eg, Canfield Scientific imaging systems) is used on which the patient's chin and forehead are secured in a fixed position, and on which a camera and flash device are mounted.[8,24] For best results, the length, color, shape, and styling of the hair must remain consistent during every photography session.[24]

Dermoscopy and videodermoscopy

Dermoscopy and videodermoscopy are noninvasive, adjunctive tools used in the diagnosis of scalp and hair disorders and guide biopsy site selection when histologic examination is warranted. These tools provide rapid visualization of subtle clinical findings not discernible on gross examination, including follicular ostia abnormalities, perifollicular skin, cutaneous blood vessels, and hair shafts.

Most handheld dermatoscopes allow for observation of the skin surface at 10-fold magnification, whereas digital dermatoscopes have working magnifications ranging from 10- to 50-fold and higher. However, handheld dermatoscopes have the advantages of being both fast and economical.[25]

Among newer handheld trichoscopes is the smartphone-compatible Handyscope created by Fotofinder, among others, which offers tremendous convenience because it attaches to the clinician's smartphone and transforms the mobile device into a digital trichoscopy tool. Videodermoscopy, although perhaps less convenient, offers certain advantages over the handheld dermoscope, because it permits rapid, high-resolution viewing at several magnifications, together with the ability to capture the viewed images digitally and to store them for later use.[8]

Trichoscopy is only useful if the clinician can interpret clinical findings. Fortunately, numerous resources are now available for trichoscopy education. In addition to textbooks, several websites, such as Dermoscopedia and Trichoscopy.net, have been developed.[26–30] Several comprehensive online learning platforms offer the advantages of being low cost, interactive, and readily accessible.

Folliscope

Folliscope (LeadM Corp, Seoul, South Korea), Medicam (FotoFinder, Bad Birnbach, Germany), and HairMetrix (Canfield Scientific, Parsippany, NJ) are noninvasive, digital image tools that capture high-resolution, real-time, magnified trichoscopy scalp imaging. These devices are composed of a handheld apparatus with a precision camera tethered to a receiving computer. The accompanying software packages determine hair density, caliber, follicular unit size, and terminal:vellus hair ratios either manually or automatically using artificial intelligence. Images can also be sent via a secure server for remote analysis.[31]

Raman Spectroscopy

Raman spectroscopy is a form of vibrational spectroscopy that provides detailed information about the state of hair, including chemical composition, interactions of molecules, and keratin structural changes, before and after treatment with products.[32] The technique is nondestructive, can be used in situ for examination of the sample, and does not require sample pretreatment.[33] Currently, the technique is typically reserved for cosmetic research because it provides detailed information about the structural modifications of hair fibers after the application of chemicals such as dyes, shampoos, and bleaches and physical procedures such as heating.[33] However, Raman spectroscopy may facilitate the diagnosis of hair disease in the future.[32]

SEMI-INVASIVE METHODS
Clinical Maneuvers

Hair pull

The hair pull is a quick, noninvasive clinical examination maneuver that identifies active hair shedding encountered in multiple etiologies, including TE and alopecia areata, among others. The test is performed ideally on hair unwashed in the previous 24 hours. After expressed permission from the patient, the examiner pulls firmly on a bundle of 50 to 60 hairs from the base of the hair shaft up through the distal terminus, sampling from at least 5 to 6 scalp areas.[34] A hair pull is generally considered positive when at least 5 to 6 hairs are released from the scalp, although a recent evidence-based analysis scrutinized this threshold as arbitrary and instead suggested a cutoff of 2 or fewer hairs, irrespective of the last hair wash.[35] Notable, false positives occur in diseases of the hair shaft such as trichorrhexis nodosa.

Modified wash test

The modified wash test helps to identify patients with TE, AGA, or both TE and AGA, and assesses the severity of shedding.[36] The test relies on the concept that in TE, only terminal hairs are shed, whereas miniaturized hairs or vellus hairs are lost in AGA.[37] For the modified wash test, patients abstain from shampooing for 5 days before testing. On the test day, patients shampoo and rinse their hair in a sink with the drain covered by gauze and then collect the hairs trapped in the gauze. The collected hairs are separated based on hair length: long hair (>5 cm) indicating terminal hairs and short hair (<3 cm) indicating vellus hairs, and counted individually.[38] The total number of shed hairs reflect the severity of hair loss (eg, TE when >100 hairs), whereas the percentage of vellus hairs indicates the severity of AGA (AGA when ≥10% vellus hairs).[39] Although this is a reliable, noninvasive test, limitations include the fact that it cannot be used in patients with very short or curly hair and it may lead to hair breakage and double counting of broken hairs.[38,40]

Imaging
Microscopy

Microscopic examination is at times required for an alopecia diagnosis. Several microscopes for clinical trichology exist, each offering their own sets of advantages. Light microscopy permits visualization of the hair shaft and determination of pigmentation, air bubbles, thickness, shape, coils, knots, invaginations, and twists.[38] Additionally, in patients with hair breakage, inspection of free ends may reveal causal qualities of hair fragility, such as tapering, weathering, cuts, and fractures.[8]

Polarized light microscopy is used typically in the diagnosis of congenital and acquired hair shaft disorders (eg, trichothiodystrophy).[41] Compared with light microscopy, polarized light is a contrast-enhancing technique to amplify and discern inner hair structure colors.[38]

Electron microscopy provides high-resolution imagery of the hair cuticle surface and permits visualization of hair shaft abnormalities and longitudinal or transversal images of the inner structures.[24] Although electron microscopy produces higher resolution images than light microscopy, the instrumentation is costly and the required hair pretreatment is extensive.[24] Additionally, electron microscopy is typically reserved for research purposes and is not used in daily dermatologic practice.[38]

Advanced microscopy devices that generate 3-dimensional (3-D) images have also been developed. For example, confocal laser scanning microscopy produces a high-resolution 3-D image of the surface structure of a hair as well as internal structures of hair.[24] The instrument enables measurements of hair shaft structures such as hair shaft thickness, specifically thickness of the medulla, cortex, and cuticle.[38,42] Atomic force microscopy produces detailed 3-D images of cuticular surfaces at the nanometer scale.[43] Although noninvasive and without sample preparation, the operator must be well-trained to accurately interpret the results.[24] Both devices are limited by the fact that they are not appropriate for daily clinical practice; however, they may be valuable for research purposes.[38]

Phototrichograms

The phototrichogram (PTG) is a minimally invasive technique that permits the in vivo analysis of the hair cycle and measurement of various hair growth parameters, including density, thickness, length, linear growth rate, and percentage of anagen and telogen hair.[44,45] To perform the PTG, hairs in a defined area are clipped 1 mm from the skin surface and photographed. The same site is photographed 2 to 3 days after the initial photograph to evaluate hair growth.[8] Conventionally, the individual hairs on both pictures on both photographs are pairwise located and compared manually.[24]

PTG technology has evolved to include advanced software for performing automated analyses. The TrichoScan (Freiburg, Germany) is operator-independent, automated software validated for the analysis of hair growth.[24,46] The program provides a precise quantification of hair loss and automated calculations of several parameters, including number of hairs, hair density, average hair length, anagen/telogen rate, number and density of vellus and terminal hair, cumulative hair thickness, and follicular units. To perform a TrichoScan analysis, a transitional area of hair loss between normal hair and a balding region is clipped.[24] The remaining hairs in the target area are dyed to increase the contrast of the hair against the skin. The target area is photographed immediately after hair dye application and days later. The TrichoScan software then analyzes the images to quickly provide accurate, reproducible measurement. Several studies have shown that compared with manually evaluated images in conventional PTG, the TrichoScan provides quicker, more reliable results.[46]

Optical coherence tomography

Optical coherence tomography is a minimally invasive imaging modality using light waves to provide highly reproducible measurements of hair shaft thickness, including the inner hair variation of diameters and shape.[24] Although optical coherence tomography may aid in the diagnosis and

monitoring of treatment response, guidelines demonstrating in vivo features of normal and alopecic scalp are in early development.[47] Ekelem and colleagues[47] recently conducted a pilot study providing an atlas, including example images and quantitative end points, of optical coherence tomography findings of both healthy and alopecia subjects. They determined that scarring alopecia is characterized by significantly increased epidermal thickness compared with nonscarring alopecia and control and decreased follicle count compared with control and nonscarring patients.[47]

INVASIVE METHODS
Scalp Biopsy

Scalp biopsy typically is performed with a cylindrical punch of at least 4 mm in diameter parallel to hair growth and is useful in equivocal cases of hair loss.[8,38] Proper location is critical for capturing relevant histologic findings rather than background androgenic alopecia. In cicatricial alopecia, trichoscopy-guided scalp biopsies should be performed within the active peripheral margins, whereas in nonscarring alopecia, a biopsy from the center of the lesion is recommended.[38] Several studies have been conducted to address the debate of horizontal versus vertical sectioning of scalp biopsies. Most recently, Palo and colleagues, in line with previous research, established that combining both horizontal and vertical sectioning of scalp biopsies maximizes the diagnostic yield when compared with either section alone.[48–50] In the case that only a single scalp biopsy is submitted, several studies found horizontal sections to be more useful in cases of noncicatricial alopecias, whereas vertical sections conferred a diagnostic advantage in cicatricial alopecias.[48–50]

SUMMARY

The early and accurate diagnosis of hair loss disorders is essential for successful management. Fortunately, a wide range of diagnostic methods are available to meet the high demand for precise, convenient, cost-effective, and minimally invasive techniques. For the practicing dermatologist, tactile assessments and direct visualization are enhanced with scoring instruments, questionnaires, handheld trichoscopy, and scalp biopsy. For research and clinical study purposes, the more precise, high-resolution tools such as videodermoscopy PTGs can be useful.

Several emerging technologies are on the horizon, but need further clinical validation. With the advent of gene expression microarray, investigators are elucidating molecular signatures of disease with the hope of better understanding etiology and predicting therapeutic response. For instance, prospectively identifying which alopecia areata patients are responsive to oral Janus Kinase (JAK) inhibitors (eg, tofacitinib) would save the time and expense associated with trials of other agents unlikely to show efficacy. Moreover, genetics may also prove useful to identify patients at risk for cicatricial alopecias, such as a predilection for central centrifugal cicatricial alopecia with *PADI3* sequence variants and expression of fibroproliferative genes.[51,52]

Patients should also be counseled on the myriad of nonclinical or unsubstantiated diagnostic tests marketed to a susceptible population motivated to find an answer for their hair loss. Although blood work can occasionally identify a nutritional deficiency or endocrine abnormality responsible for hair loss, these tests are not necessary for most patients and should only be ordered when supporting clinical evidence is present. Mass spectrometry of hair shafts, gut microbiome analysis, and elaborate serologic metabolic assessments, among others, are expensive efforts that may cloud rather than inform a diagnosis.

CLINICS CARE POINTS

- Hair and scalp diagnoses are made with tactile assessments and direct visualization, which are further enhanced with scoring instruments, questionnaires, handheld trichoscopy, and scalp biopsy.
- For research and clinical study purposes, the more precise, high-resolution tools such as videodermoscopy PTGs, electron microscopy, and atomic force microscopy can be useful.
- Patients should be counseled on the abundance of nonclinical or unsubstantiated diagnostic tests marketed to a susceptible population motivated to find an answer for their hair loss as these tests can often cloud, rather than inform diagnosis.

REFERENCES

1. Wilmer EN, Gustafson CJ, Ahn CS, et al. Most common dermatologic conditions encountered by dermatologists and nondermatologists. Cutis 2014; 94(6):285–92.
2. Shapiro J, Otberg N. Hair loss and restoration. Boca raton, FL: CRC Press; 2015.
3. Barber B, Kaufman K, Kozloff R, et al. A hair growth questionnaire for use in the evaluation of therapeutic effects in men. J Dermatol Treat 1998;9(3):181–6.
4. Harness J, Mamolo C, Olsen E, et al. The women's hair growth questionnaire: development and validation of a patient-reported measure for treatment efficacy in androgenetic alopecia. In: Paper presented at: journal of the American Academy of Dermatology. 2009.
5. Marks DH, Penzi LR, Ibler E, et al. The medical and psychosocial associations of alopecia: recognizing hair loss as more than a cosmetic concern. Am J Clin Dermatol 2019;20(2):195–200.
6. Fischer TW, Schmidt S, Strauss B, et al. [Hairdex: a tool for evaluation of disease-specific quality of life in patients with hair diseases]. Hautarzt 2001;52(3):219–27.
7. Trüeb RM. The difficult hair loss patient: guide to successful management of alopecia and related conditions. Cham: Springer; 2015.
8. Dhurat R, Saraogi P. Hair evaluation methods: merits and demerits. Int J Trichol 2009;1(2):108–19.
9. Wasko CA, Mackley CL, Sperling LC, et al. Standardizing the 60-second hair count. Arch Dermatol 2008;144(6):759–62.
10. Piraccini BM. Evaluation of hair loss. In: Ioannides D, Tosti A, editors. Alopeciaspractical evaluation and management, vol 47. Basel: Karger Publishers; 2015. p. 10–20.
11. Jackson AJ, Price VH. How to diagnose hair loss. Dermatol Clin 2013;31(1):21–8.
12. Sinclair R, Torkamani N, Jones L. Androgenetic alopecia: new insights into the pathogenesis and mechanism of hair loss. F1000Res 2015;4(F1000 Faculty Rev):585.
13. Martínez-Velasco MA, Vázquez-Herrera NE, Maddy AJ, et al. The hair shedding visual scale: a quick tool to assess hair loss in women. Dermatol Ther (Heidelb) 2017;7(1):155–65.
14. Norwood OT. Incidence of female androgenetic alopecia (female pattern alopecia). Dermatol Surg 2001;27(1):53–4.
15. Olsen EA. Female pattern hair loss. J Am Acad Dermatol 2001;45(3):S70–80.
16. Gupta M, Mysore V. Classifications of patterned hair loss: a review. J Cutan Aesthet Surg 2016;9(1):3.
17. Harries M, Tosti A, Bergfeld W, et al. Towards a consensus on how to diagnose and quantify female pattern hair loss–The 'Female Pattern Hair Loss Severity Index (FPHL-SI)'. J Eur Acad Dermatol Venereol 2016;30(4):667–76.
18. Olsen EA, Hordinsky MK, Price VH, et al. Alopecia areata investigational assessment guidelines–Part II. J Am Acad Dermatol 2004;51(3):440–7.
19. Olsen EA, Canfield D. SALT II: a new take on the Severity of Alopecia Tool (SALT) for determining percentage scalp hair loss. J Am Acad Dermatol 2016; 75(6):1268–70.
20. Bernardis E, Castelo-Soccio L. Quantifying alopecia areata via texture analysis to automate the salt score computation. In: Paper presented at: Journal of investigative dermatology symposium proceedings. 2018.

21. Chiang C, Sah D, Cho BK, et al. Hydroxychloroquine and lichen planopilaris: efficacy and introduction of Lichen Planopilaris Activity Index scoring system. J Am Acad Dermatol 2010;62(3):387–92.

22. Sperling LC, Nguyen JV. Commentary: treatment of lichen planopilaris: some progress, but a long way to go. J Am Acad Dermatol 2010;62(3):398–401.

23. Saceda-Corralo D, Moreno-Arrones ÓM, Fonda-Pascual P, et al. Development and validation of the frontal fibrosing alopecia severity score. J Am Acad Dermatol 2018;78(3):522–9.

24. Blume-Peytavi U, Hillmann K, Guarrera M. Hair growth assessment techniques. In: Blume-Peytavi U, Tosti A, Trüeb RM, editors. Hair growth and disorders. London: Springer; 2008. p. 125–57.

25. Mubki T, Rudnicka L, Olszewska M, et al. Evaluation and diagnosis of the hair loss patient: part II. Trichoscopic and laboratory evaluations. J Am Acad Dermatol 2014;71(3). 431. e431-431. e411.

26. Trichoscopy.net. Sukhdeo medical, PLLC. Available at: https://www.trichoscopy.net/. Accessed 20 October, 2020.

27. Dermoscopedia. International dermoscopy society 2020. Available at: https://dermoscopedia.org/Main_Page. Accessed 20 Oct, 2020.

28. Tosti A. Dermoscopy of the hair and nails. Boca raton, FL: CRC Press; 2015.

29. Rudnicka L, Olszewska M, Rakowska A. Atlas of trichoscopy: dermoscopy in hair and scalp disease. London: Springer Science & Business Media; 2012.

30. Malakar S. Trichoscopy: a text and atlas. New Delhi: JP Medical Ltd; 2017.

31. Lee BSL, Chan J-YL, Monselise A, et al. Assessment of hair density and caliber in Caucasian and Asian female subjects with female pattern hair loss by using the Folliscope. J Am Acad Dermatol 2012;66(1):166.

32. Zhang G, Senak L, Moore DJ. Measuring changes in chemistry, composition, and molecular structure within hair fibers by infrared and Raman spectroscopic imaging. J Biomed Opt 2011;16(5):056009.

33. dos Santos JD, Edwards HG, de Oliveira LFC. Raman spectroscopy and electronic microscopy structural studies of Caucasian and Afro human hair. Heliyon 2019;5(5):e01582.

34. Shapiro J, Wiseman M, Lui H. Practical management of hair loss. Can Fam Physician 2000;46(7):1469–77.

35. McDonald KA, Shelley AJ, Colantonio S, et al. Hair pull test: evidence-based update and revision of guidelines. J Am Acad Dermatol 2017;76(3):472–7.

36. Guarrera M, Fiorucci MC, Rebora A. Methods of hair loss evaluation: a comparison of T richo S can® with the modified wash test. Exp Dermatol 2013;22(7):482–4.

37. Guarrera M, Rebora A. Hair evaluation method: pull test and wash test. Agache's Measuring Skin 2017;115:827–30.

38. Hillmann K, Blume-Peytavi U. Diagnosis of hair disorders. In: Paper presented at: seminars in cutaneous medicine and surgery. 2009.

39. Rebora A, Guarrera M, Baldari M, et al. Distinguishing androgenetic alopecia from chronic telogen effluvium when associated in the same patient: a simple noninvasive method. Arch Dermatol 2005;141(10):1243–5.

40. Guarrera M, Cardo P, Rebora A. Assessing the reliability of the Modified Wash Test. G Ital Dermatol Venereol 2011;146(4):289–94.

41. Humbert P, Fanian F, Maibach H. Agache's measuring the skin. Cham: Springer International Publishing; 2019.

42. Rudnicka L, Olszewska M, Rakowska A. In vivo reflectance confocal microscopy: usefulness for diagnosing hair diseases. J Dermatol Case Rep 2008;2(4):55.

43. Seshadri IP, Bhushan B. In situ tensile deformation characterization of human hair with atomic force microscopy. Acta Materialia 2008;56(4):774–81.

44. Reygagne P. Phototrichogram. In: Humbert P, Fanian F, Maibach HI, et al, editors. Agache's measuring the skin: non-invasive investigations, physiology, normal constants. Cham: Springer International Publishing; 2017. p. 813–25.

45. Brancato S, Cartigliani C, Bonfigli A, et al. Quantitative analysis using the phototrichogram technique of an Italian Population Suffering from Androgenic Alopecia. Cosmetics 2018;5(2):28.

46. Gassmueller J, Rowold E, Frase T, et al. Validation of TrichoScan® technology as a fully-automated tool for evaluation of hair growth parameters. Eur J Dermatol 2009;19(3):224–31.

47. Ekelem C, Feil N, Csuka E, et al. Optical coherence tomography in the evaluation of the scalp and hair: common features and clinical utility. Lasers Surg Med 2020;53(1):129–40.

48. Palo S, Biligi DS. Utility of horizontal and vertical sections of scalp biopsies in various forms of primary alopecias. J Lab physicians 2018;10(1):95.

49. Özcan D, Özen Ö, Seçkin D. Vertical vs. transverse sections of scalp biopsy specimens: a pilot study on the comparison of the diagnostic value of two techniques in alopecia. Clin Exp Dermatol Clin Dermatol 2011;36(8):855–63.

50. Elston DM, Ferringer T, Dalton S, et al. A comparison of vertical versus transverse sections in the evaluation of alopecia biopsy specimens. J Am Acad Dermatol 2005;53(2):267–72.

51. Aguh C, Dina Y, Talbot CC Jr, et al. Fibroproliferative genes are preferentially expressed in central centrifugal cicatricial alopecia. J Am Acad Dermatol 2018;79(5):904–12.e901.

52. Malki L, Sarig O, Romano M-T, et al. Variant PADI3 in central centrifugal cicatricial alopecia. N Engl J Med 2019;380(9):833–41.

Scarring Alopecia
Diagnosis and New Treatment Options

Maria Hordinsky, MD

KEYWORDS

- Cicatricial alopecia • Scarring hair loss • Stem cells

KEY POINTS

- Review of the primary cicatricial alopecias.
- Current and evolving treatments and research.
- Pathogenesis of CCCA not well understood; inciting factors are unclear there are no established treatment guideline.

The primary cicatricial alopecias are a heterogeneous group of diseases that have the common end of follicular scarring. Scarring results from the loss of follicular stem cells and the inflammatory destruction of the hair follicle and sebaceous glands. The primary cicatricial alopecias are subdivided by the type of inflammation detected on histologic examination and are described as lymphocytic or neutrophilic or mixed.[1] The more common lymphocytic cicatricial alopecias include:

- Central centrifugal scarring alopecia
- Discoid lupus erythematosus
- Frontal fibrosing alopecia
- Lichen planopilaris

Alopecia mucinosa, keratosis follicularis spinulosa decalvans, and pseudopelade of Brocq are also considered to be lymphocytic cicatricial alopecias but are not as common. Pseudopelade of Brocq is also a subject of debate, because this entity is thought by many clinicians to be a late stage of lichen planopilaris and not a separate entity.

The more common neutrophilic cicatricial alopecias include:

- Folliculitis decalvans
- Dissecting cellulitis

Examples of mixed cicatricial alopecias include:

- Acne keloidalis
- Acne necrotica
- Erosive pustular dermatoses, an idiopathic, chronic, relapsing pustular dermatosis of the scalp that is frequently preceded by a history of trauma

PATHOGENESIS OF THE CICATRICIAL ALOPECIAS

There are several hypotheses as to why cicatricial alopecias occur. These hypotheses include the loss of follicular immune privilege, changes in the local pilosebaceous unit microbiome, abnormal lipid metabolism, and a potential role for mast cells, particularly in the lymphocytic cicatricial alopecias. The loss of immune privilege occurs in the hair follicle bulge region, the location of hair follicle stem cells. The collapse of this region has been associated with increased expression of major histocompatibility class I and II, reduced CD200 expression, and increased expression of chemokine (C-X-C motif) ligands (CXCL1 CXCL9/CXCL10/CXCL11), all of which lead to permanent damage of hair follicle stem cells. The role of genetics in the cicatricial alopecias is still unfolding. Allergic contact dermatitis to chemicals as in hair care products has also been associated with a lymphocytic cicatricial alopecia.[2,3]

Department of Dermatology, University of Minnesota, 516 Delaware Street Southeast, MMC 98, Minneapolis, MN 55455, USA
E-mail address: hordi001@umn.edu

Dermatol Clin 39 (2021) 383–388
https://doi.org/10.1016/j.det.2021.05.001

PATIENT EVALUATION OVERVIEW

It is important to recognize that patients who present with cicatricial alopecia may also have an associated nonscarring alopecia, such as androgenetic alopecia or telogen effluvium. Therefore, the history needs to be as thorough as it would be for any patient presenting with the chief complaint of hair loss. Patients need to be queried on many topics, including the following[4–6]:

- Hair care habits
- Duration of the hair disease
- Disease activity: is it worsening or stable?
- Prescription and nonprescription medications
- Symptoms: pain, itch, burning, whether there is a hair care product relationship
- Eyebrow, eyelash, and body hair: is there too much or too little?
- Nail abnormalities
- Use of supplements, herbals/botanicals
- Family history of hair diseases
- Signs of androgen excess
- History of autoimmune/endocrine diseases
- Recent or chronic illnesses
- Recent surgical procedures
- For women, query about the menstrual cycle/pregnancies

PATIENT EXAMINATION

The examination should focus on assessing the presence or absence of the following and, if applicable, the use of trichoscopy:

- Scale, erythema, folliculitis, scarring, or atrophy in affected hair-bearing areas
- Eyebrow, eyelash, or body hair loss
- Nail abnormalities
- Findings of androgen excess
- Vellus, indeterminate, and terminal fibers ideally using scoring systems such as the Ludwig or Hamilton-Norwood classification systems, the Severity of Alopecia Scoring Tool (SALT score), or the Lichen Planopilaris Activity Index (LPPAI)

Trichoscopy, or dermoscopy of the scalp, can complement the clinical examination and is usually performed with a handheld dermatoscope (10× magnification) or with a videodermoscope (up to 1000× magnification). The instrument is directly applied to the scalp to better examine follicular ostia, perifollicular scale and erythema, vasculature, and hair shafts. The absence of follicular ostia suggests a cicatricial alopecia, as does the presence of white dots, which are characteristic of fibrosis. Black dots, which can indicate destroyed or broken hair fibers at the level of the scalp, may be seen in patients with dissecting cellulitis. Yellow dots can be present on the scalp of patients with discoid lupus erythematosus but can also be seen in those with alopecia areata or pattern hair loss. A honeycomb pigmented network of brown, regularly sized meshes encircling hypopigmented areas can be seen in patients with central centrifugal cicatricial alopecia.

If making a diagnosis of cicatricial alopecia is challenging, a scalp biopsy can be obtained to confirm the diagnosis.[7] Ideally, the biopsy should be taken from a hair-bearing areas with signs of active inflammation and positive hair-pull test. Biopsying areas of complete alopecia is usually avoided but, if there is interest in assessing how much scarring has occurred, a biopsy from such a region may be helpful to assess the degree of scarring. Some clinicians use dermoscopy to guide them to the most active site to biopsy. The gold standard is to take 2 4-mm punch biopsies because this allows for evaluation of hair follicles and inflammation in both vertical and horizontal sections. The biopsy report will then not only confirm the diagnosis but examination of horizontal sections will provide additional information on the number of viable follicles and extent of the inflammatory process. Such information gives the clinician more data to share with the patient and may help with setting treatment expectations. Recent research also suggests that normal-appearing scalp may not be normal. Studies have shown follicular inflammation in clinically noninvolved scalp in both the neutrophilic and lymphocytic alopecias. This finding has led to the suggestion that the treatments should be focused not only on visible lesions but on the entire scalp.

Of note, there are no required blood tests for patients with cicatricial alopecias. Bacterial cultures may be beneficial if the pustular component does not respond to standard treatment. In some cases, a scalp biopsy for tissue culture may also be needed, such as when the patient is not responding to standard therapies. *Staphylococcus aureus* is commonly found on tissue culture examination.

Many patients with a cicatricial alopecia report scalp pain, tenderness, burning, or pruritus. Some patients with lichen planopilaris even describe their scalp as being on fire. This symptom may be related to the stem cell region of the hair follicle that is under attack being heavily innervated. It is postulated that there may be a component of neurogenic inflammation present in patients with scalp symptoms and it has been suggested that topical or oral gabapentin may be beneficial for such patients.[8]

CLINICAL
Lymphocytic Primary Cicatricial Alopecias

Lichen planopilaris, frontal fibrosing alopecia, and central centrifugal cicatricial alopecia are the most common lymphocytic primary cicatricial alopecias. Discoid lupus erythematosus is also fairly common, but entities such as alopecia mucinosa, pseudopelade of Brocq, and keratosis follicularis spinulosa decalvans are considered to be less common.

Alopecia mucinosa
This lymphocytic primary cicatricial alopecia is also known as follicular mucinosis.[9] Permanent hair loss occurs because of hair follicles being replaced by mucin. Developing alopecia mucinosa can be idiopathic or associated with cutaneous T-cell lymphoma.

Central centrifugal cicatricial alopecia
This entity primarily affects women of African descent, occurs on the crown of the scalp, and moves in a centrifugal pattern to the parietal scalp.[10] Central centrifugal cicatricial alopecia is discussed in more detail in a separate article in this issue.

Discoid lupus erythematosus
Discoid lupus erythematosus may occur in the absence of any systemic disease or in association with systemic lupus erythematosus.[11] Lesions are characterized as well-demarcated plaques with central hyperkeratosis, telangiectasia, hypopigmentation, and hyperpigmentation.

Keratosis follicularis spinulosa decalvans
Keratosis follicularis spinulosa decalvans is considered a rare genetic disorder that first presents in infancy with follicular papules and keratotic spines.[12] A mutation in the membrane-bound transcription factor proteases site 2 gene on the X chromosome has been identified.

Lichen planopilaris
Lichen planopilaris is considered a follicular variant of lichen planus and presents with perifollicular erythema and hyperkeratosis, usually at the periphery of lesions, in contrast with discoid lupus erythematosus, where disease activity is more centrally located.[13]

Frontal fibrosing alopecia
Frontal fibrosing alopecia is discussed in greater detail in a separate article in this issue but, in brief, this is considered to be an emerging disease characterized by a bandlike alopecia that affects the frontal scalp.[14] Follicular hyperkeratosis and perifollicular erythema are commonly seen at the leading edge. Loss of eyebrow fibers is common, as is the presence of follicular-based flesh-colored papules in the temporal region. Vein prominence in the affected forehead/frontal scalp region may also be seen.

Pseudopelade of Brocq
As mentioned earlier, some clinicians view this entity, which is characterized by the clinical appearance of small skin-colored patches of alopecia looking like footprints in the snow, to be a late stage of lichen planopilaris.[15]

Neutrophilic Primary Cicatricial Alopecia

Dissecting cellulitis of the scalp
This entity is also called perifolliculitis capitis abscedens et suffodiens of Hoffman and can occur alone or in association with hidradenitis suppurativa or acne conglobata. Follicular papules, pustules, nodules, and abscesses form on the scalp in affected patients.[16]

Folliculitis decalvans
Folliculitis decalvans is characterized by inflamed papules, pustules, and follicular hyperkeratosis and usually starts on the vertex of the scalp.[17] Tufted folliculitis, described as multiple hair fibers emerging from a single follicle, is commonly seen.

Mixed

Acne keloidalis nuchae
Acne keloidalis nuchae occurs primarily in black men and is characterized by dome-shaped follicular papules, pustules, and plaques on the occipital scalp. This entity is thought to be related to trauma.[18]

Acne necrotica
This disease is considered to be a rare entity and is characterized by the development of papules on the scalp that undergo necrosis and resolution characterized by poxlike scars.[19]

Erosive pustular dermatosis of the scalp
Affected patients present with pustules, erosions, and crusted plaques that developed after trauma or surgery on the scalp or after treatment of actinic keratosis.[20]

TREATMENT

The goals of treatment are to arrest or slow disease progression and to reduce symptoms. Although some hair regrowth can occur in sites of alopecia where there has not been permanent injury, hair will not regrow from follicles that have been permanently damaged by a cicatricial alopecia process. Beginning treatment early is important to ensure the likelihood of disease arrest and possible scalp hair regrowth. Stabilization of the disease process may be considered a successful outcome.

LYMPHOCYTIC CICATRICIAL ALOPECIAS

The choice of treatment of the lymphocytic cicatricial alopecias is usually based on clinical activity, severity of symptoms, and disease activity. Treatments are generally grouped into 3 tiers of disease severity: patients with limited active disease, moderate disease, or severe disease.[21–23]

- Tier 1 treatments for patients with limited active disease include use of topical high-potency corticosteroids, intralesional steroids, or topical nonsteroid antiinflammatory creams such as tacrolimus or pimecrolimus.
- Tier 2 treatments for patients with moderate disease include hydroxychloroquine, low-dose oral antibiotics for their antiinflammatory effect or specific antimicrobial effect, or acitretin.
- Tier 3 treatments include immunosuppressive medications such as cyclosporine, prednisone, or mycophenolate mofetil.

Recent research has identified lipid metabolism abnormalities involving peroxisomes and peroxisome proliferator-activated receptor gamma (PPAR-γ) in the lymphocytic cicatricial alopecias and, in particular, lichen planopilaris. This finding has led some clinicians to prescribe drugs such as pioglitazone hydrochloride, with variable success. Likewise, Janus kinase (JAK) inhibitors such as the pan-JAK inhibitor, tofacitinib, are emerging as novel treatment options for many immune-mediated and inflammatory diseases in dermatology, including the lymphocytic cicatricial alopecias. More clinical research will be forthcoming on the efficacy of this approach. Once disease activity has stabilized, hair regrowth agents may be prescribed. These agents include topical and oral minoxidil as well as finasteride and, in some cases, photobiomodulation.

NEUTROPHILIC CICATRICIAL ALOPECIAS

For patients experiencing a neutrophilic cicatricial alopecia, pustules should be cultured and antibiotic sensitivities determined. The use of retinoids may or may not be helpful and, in some cases, addition of prednisone may improve efficacy. Oral L-tyrosine administration, laser hair removal, and intranasal eradication of S aureus are other recommendations. Intralesional corticosteroid injections can also be

helpful with stabilizing disease activity. Case reports of tumor necrosis factor (TNF) alpha injections being beneficial in the management of neutrophilic cicatricial alopecias have been published, but there are also case reports of scarring alopecias occurring in patients receiving a TNF alpha biologic.[24–26]

Patients experiencing a mixed type of cicatricial alopecia can be prescribed any combination of those recommended for the lymphocytic or neutrophilic cicatricial alopecias.

Cosmetic recommendations may also be helpful to patients with a cicatricial alopecia. Changes in hairstyling techniques, wearing hair pieces or wigs, or applying cosmetics to assist in camouflaging hair loss may be beneficial. Hair transplant can be considered but should only be done if the disease is quiet.[27]

Validated scales to measure disease extent, activity, and treatment response are being developed for some of the cicatricial alopecias. One validated scale that is currently available is LPPAI score.[28] This score provides a standardized measure that takes into account both patient symptoms and clinical features and is calculated from 3 subjective factors (pruritus, pain, burning) as well as 5 objective factors (erythema, perifollicular erythema, perifollicular scale, anagen pull test, and spreading). These factors are each assigned a score, with 0 = absent, 1 = mild, 2 = moderate, and 3 = severe. The first 3 factors are as reported by the patient and the next 3 factors are evaluated by the dermatologist based on clinical examination. The anagen pull test is evaluated as either 0 = negative or 1 = positive. Spreading is evaluated as 0 = no spreading, 1 = undetermined, 2 = spreading. Each factor is weighted differently to reflect accuracy and precision; the anagen pull test is given the most weight because it is the most objective and reproducible factor, whereas the symptomatic factors are given the least weight because they are most subjective. The LPPAI calculation is as follows, and can be used longitudinally to monitor disease activity and treatment responses:

LPPAI = (pruritus + pain + burning)/3 + (scalp erythema + perifollicular erythema + perifollicular scale)/3 + 2.5(pull test) + 1.5 (spreading/2)

FUTURE

Clinical and basic science investigations are now focusing primarily on the following cicatricial alopecias: lichen planopilaris, frontal fibrosing alopecia, and central centrifugal cicatricial alopecia. Transcriptome, lipidome, and other new technologies, as well as the use of genetically engineered mouse models, are providing new insight into the pathogenesis of these diseases. Genetic studies continue as well, with the most progress made with frontal fibrosing alopecia and central centrifugal cicatricial alopecia, where a recent genome-wide association study showed a significant association with frontal fibrosing alopecia at 4 genomic loci: 2p22.2, 6p21.1, 8q24.22, and 15q2.1. Fine mapping within the 2p22.2 and 6p21.1 loci revealed associations with a presumed causal missense variant in CYP1B1, which encodes a member of the cytochrome P450 family, and the HLA-B*07:02 allele, respectively, suggesting that frontal fibrosing alopecia is a genetically predisposed disorder in inflammatory and immune responses. A variant of PADI3 has been found in central centrifugal cicatricial alopecia via whole-exome sequencing, suggesting that this mutation may result in improper formation of hair shaft, leading to the central centrifugal cicatricial alopecia phenotype. Gene expression profiling has also shown decreased tissue expression of PPAR-γ in lichen planopilaris lesions compared with unaffected skin, suggesting that lichen planopilaris might be characterized by dysregulated fatty acid and/or glucose metabolism. The finding that mammalian target of rapamycin (mTOR) signaling pathway proteins, which are central regulators of cell metabolism, show altered expression in the hair follicles of lichen planopilaris and frontal fibrosing alopecia patients compared with those of healthy controls also supports this observation.[2,29–32]

Future directions identified at a Cicatricial Alopecia Research Foundation meeting held in conjunction with an annual meeting of the Society of Investigative Dermatology include standardizing sample collection methods and patient information with the goal of having good-quality samples for RNA sequencing, transcriptomics, lipidomics, proteomics, and new technologies as they become available. Another goal is to access high-end computational analyses to deconvolute the immune infiltrate signals and to predict druggable candidates for the various types of primary cicatricial alopecias. The bacteria, viruses, and fungi that inhabit the skin and gut also have to be included in investigations of the primary cicatricial alopecias.

CLINICS CARE POINTS

- Data are limited on the treatment of CCCA, and there are no established treatment guidelines.

- For patients with mild CCCA initial treatment with a high-potency topical corticosteroid is recommended.
- For patients with more extensive disease we suggest the inclusion of an oral tetracycline-class antibiotic.

DISCLOSURE

The author is a member of the Board of Directors, Cicatricial Alopecia Research Foundation (CARF).

REFERENCES

1. Ross EK, Tan E, Shapiro J. Update on primary cicatricial alopecias. J Am Acad Dermatol 2005;53(3):1–37.
2. Sundberg JP, Hordinsky M, Bergfeld W, et al. Cicatricial alopecia research foundation meeting. May 2016: progress toward the diagnosis, treatment and care of primary cicatricial alopecias. Exp Dermatol 2018;27(3):302–10.
3. Prasad S, Marks DH, Burns LJ, et al. Patch testing and contact allergen avoidance in patients with lichen planopilaris and/or frontal fibrosing alopecia: a cohort study. J Am Acad Dermatol 2020;83(2):659–61.
4. Mubki T, Rudnicka L, Olszewska M, et al. Evaluation and diagnosis of the hair loss patient: part I. History and clinical examination. J Am Acad Dermatol 2014;71(3):415.e1–15.
5. Mubki T, Rudnicka L, Olszewska M, et al. Evaluation and diagnosis of the hair loss patient: part II. Trichoscopic and laboratory evaluations. J Am Acad Dermatol 2014;71(3):431.e1–11.
6. Lacarrubba F, Micali G, Tosti A. Scalp dermoscopy or trichoscopy. Curr Probl Dermatol 2015;47:21–32.
7. Starace M, Orlando G, Alessandrini A, et al. Diffuse variants of scalp lichen planopilaris: clinical, trichoscopic, and histopathologic features of 40 patients. J Am Acad Dermatol 2020;83(6):1659–67.
8. Doche I, Wilcox GL, Ericson M, et al. Evidence for neurogenic inflammation in lichen planopilaris and frontal fibrosing alopecia pathogenic mechanism. Exp Dermatol 2020;29(3):282–5.
9. Zvulunov A, Shkalim V, Ben-Amitai D, et al. Clinical and histopathologic spectrum of alopecia mucinosa/follicular mucinosis and its natural history in children. J Am Acad Dermatol 2012;67:1174.
10. Summers P, Kyei A, Bergfeld W. Central centrifugal cicatricial alopecia - an approach to diagnosis and management. Int J Dermatol 2011;50:1457.
11. Hordinsky M. Cicatricial alopecia: discoid lupus erythematosus. Dermatol Ther 2008;21(4):245–8.

12. Castori M, Covaciu C, Paradisi M, et al. Clinical and genetic heterogeneity in keratosis follicularis spinulosa decalvans. Eur J Med Genet 2009;52:53.

13. Kang H, Alzolibani AA, Otberg N, et al. Lichen planopilaris. Dermatol Ther 2008;21:249.

14. Ho A, Shapiro J. Medical therapy for frontal fibrosing alopecia: a review and clinical approach. J Am Acad Dermatol 2019;81(2):568–80.

15. Bergner T, Braun-Falco O. Pseudopelade of Brocq. J Am Acad Dermatol 1991;25(5 Pt 1):865–6.

16. Scheinfeld NS. A case of dissecting cellulitis and a review of the literature. Dermatol Online J 2003;9:8.

17. Powell JJ, Dawber RP, Gatter K. Folliculitis decalvans including tufted folliculitis: clinical, histological and therapeutic findings. Br J Dermatol 1999;140:328.

18. George AO, Akanji AO, Nduka EU, et al. Clinical, biochemical and morphologic features of acne keloidalis in a black population. Int J Dermatol 1993;32:714.

19. Kossard S, Collins A, McCrossin I. Necrotizing lymphocytic folliculitis: the early lesion of acne necrotica (varioliformis). J Am Acad Dermatol 1987;16:1007.

20. Starace M, Loi C, Bruni F, et al. Erosive pustular dermatosis of the scalp: Clinical, trichoscopic, and histopathologic features of 20 cases. J Am Acad Dermatol 2017;76:1109.

21. Price VH. The medical treatment of cicatricial alopecia. Semin Cutan Med Surg 2006;25:56.

22. Mesinkovska NA, Tellez A, Dawes D, et al. The use of oral pioglitazone in the treatment of lichen planopilaris. J Am Acad Dermatol 2015;72:355.

23. Yang CC, Khanna T, Sallee B, et al. Tofacitinib for the treatment of lichen planopilaris: a case series. Dermatol Ther 2018;31(6):e12656.

24. Rambhia PH, Conic RRZ, Murad A, et al. Updates in therapeutics for folliculitis decalvans: a systematic review with evidence-based analysis. J Am Acad Dermatol 2019;3:794–801.e1.

25. Thomas J, Aguh C. Approach to treatment of refractory dissecting cellulitis of the scalp: a systematic review. J Dermatolog Treat 2021;32(2):144–9.

26. Bolduc C, Sperling LC, Shapiro J. Primary cicatricial alopecia: Other lymphocytic primary cicatricial alopecias and neutrophilic and mixed primary cicatricial alopecias. J Am Acad Dermatol 2016;75(6):1101–17.

27. Chiang C, Sah D, Cho BK, et al. Hydroxychloroquine and lichen planopilaris: efficacy and introduction of Lichen Planopilaris Activity Index scoring system. J Am Acad Dermatol 2010;62:387.

28. Donovan JC, Shapiro RL, Shapiro P, et al. A review of scalp camouflaging agents and prostheses for individuals with hair loss. Dermatol Online J 2012;18:1.

29. Hobo A, Harada K, Maeda T, et al. IL-17-positive mast cell infiltration in the lesional skin of lichen planopilaris: possible role of mast cells in inducing inflammation and dermal fibrosis in cicatricial alopecia. Exp Dermatol 2020;29(3):273–7.

30. Tziotzios C, Petridis C, Dand N, et al. Genome-wide association study in frontal fibrosing alopecia identifies four susceptibility loci including HLA-B*07:02. Nat Commun 2019;10:1150.

31. Malki L, Sarig O, Romano MT, et al. Variant PADI3 in central centrifugal cicatricial alopecia. N Engl J Med 2019;380:833.

32. Dicle O, Celik-Ozenci C, Sahin P, et al. Differential expression of mTOR signaling pathway proteins in lichen planopilaris and frontal fibrosing alopecia. Acta Histochem 2018;120:837.

Central Centrifugal Cicatricial Alopecia
Challenges and Treatments

Christina N. Lawson, MD[a],*, Awa Bakayoko, BA[b], Valerie D. Callender, MD[c]

KEYWORDS

• Central centrifugal cicatricial alopecia • CCCA • Scarring alopecia • Hair restoration • Treatment

KEY POINTS

- Central centrifugal cicatricial alopecia (CCCA) is the most common form of primary scarring alopecia in women of African descent.
- At the molecular level, an autosomal dominant mode of inheritance, mutations in protein *PADI3*, and upregulation of critical fibroproliferative genes have all been linked to patients with CCCA.
- CCCA often occurs in the absence of clinical signs of overt inflammation and instead fibrosis is often the predominant feature.
- The presence of a white/gray peripilar follicular halo on dermoscopy is both sensitive and specific for CCCA and should be followed up with biopsy for confirmatory diagnosis.
- Treatment of CCCA can be divided into 2 stages (anti-inflammatory phase and regrowth phase) and more published case-controlled studies are needed.

INTRODUCTION

Central centrifugal cicatricial alopecia (CCCA) is a progressive, inflammatory scarring alopecia that primarily affects women of African descent and rarely men. Since its original description in 1968, the current term CCCA has replaced the older nomenclature that included "hot comb alopecia,"[1] "follicular degeneration syndrome,"[2] and "chemically induced scarring alopecia."[3] The term CCCA was created by the North American Hair Research Society[4] to provide a more accurate clinicopathologic description.

PREVALENCE

The true prevalence of CCCA has yet to be established; however, multiple studies have been conducted to explore the prevalence in different demographics. A study completed in 2011 sought to discern the prevalence of CCCA in African American women, where patients from the central/southeast United States were recruited and their hair loss evaluated through the use of a standardized photographic scale[5] and questionnaire; the study concluded a prevalence of 5.6% in a study of 529 subjects.[6,7] A different 2011 population study conducted in Cleveland, Ohio, surveyed black women in their community for hair loss using the same photographic scale and found that 28% of the patients exhibited clinical hair loss grade (CHLG) of 2 or higher and 59% of patients within this group received a CHLG of 3 to 5, bringing a projected prevalence in this study to roughly 16%.[8] A study completed in Cape Town, South Africa, found the prevalence of CCCA to be 2.7% in African women, with the prevalence increasing to 6.7% in African women older than 50 years.[9]

The difference in reported prevalence is likely due to a multitude of factors, including cultural elements, presence of systemic disease, age, hair

[a] Dermatology Associates of Lancaster, 1650 Crooked Oak Drive, Suite 200, Lancaster, PA 17601, USA; [b] Lewis Katz School of Medicine, Temple University, 3500 North Broad Street, Philadelphia, PA 19140, USA; [c] Callender Dermatology and Cosmetic Center, 12200 Annapolis Road, Suite 315, Glenn Dale, MD 20769, USA
* Corresponding author. Callender Dermatology and Cosmetic Center, 12200 Annapolis Road, Suite 315, Glenn Dale, MD 20769, USA
E-mail address: clawson2011@gmail.com

Dermatol Clin 39 (2021) 389–405
https://doi.org/10.1016/j.det.2021.03.004

grooming practices, and genetics. However, a limitation to many of these studies involves the sole use of a photographic scale, without a biopsy-proven diagnosis of CCCA. More studies must be conducted to tease out the true prevalence in the adult female population.

Other demographics also can be affected by CCCA; however, this is on a much smaller scale. Although rare in children, investigators have reported biopsy-proven CCCA pediatric cases in the literature.[10] CCCA has also been reported in male individuals of African descent[11] and it is critical to differentiate this from androgenetic alopecia (AGA).[12]

PATHOGENESIS

The pathogenesis of CCCA is believed to involve a complex mixture of a multitude of factors including but not limited to genetic predisposition,[13] variants in gene expression,[14] ethnic hair care practices,[15] and disruption of the balance between proinflammatory and anti-inflammatory factors. One study of 14 South African index families with 31 immediate family members found evidence to suggest that CCCA can be inherited in an autosomal dominant fashion.[13]

New research[14] suggests that pathogenic variations in the gene encoding peptidyl arginine deiminase type III (PADI3) have been implicated in the pathogenesis of CCCA. PADI3 is an enzyme responsible for the posttranslational deimination of proteins crucial in hair shaft formation. Missense and splice site mutations located in highly conserved regions of the PADI3 gene were found to be higher among patients with CCCA than in control groups of women of African descent ($P = .002$).[14] These mutations likely lead to the creation of a pathogenic protein product that would be subject to protein misfolding, destruction, and/or sequestration creating fragile hair shafts that can be subject to easy breakage.

CCCA is also characterized by low-grade inflammation with subsequent progression to fibrosis. Upregulation of fibroproliferative genes such as platelet-derived growth factor (PDGF), collagen gene I and III (COL I and COL III), and matrix metallopeptidase genes 1, 2, and 7 (MMP1, MMP2, MMP7) have been identified in patients with CCCA.[16]

ASSOCIATED FINDINGS

More recent literature has explored the possible connection between CCCA and systemic diseases. One study reported a statistically significant increase in the prevalence of diabetes mellitus type 2 among patients with CCCA, suggesting that CCCA may be a marker of metabolic dysregulation.[8] A retrospective study reported that women with CCCA were found to have a nearly 5 times increased odds of having uterine leiomyomas compared with race-matched, age-matched, and sex-matched controls.[17] This association between uterine leiomyomas with CCCA further supports the notion that fibroproliferative genes play an important role in the pathogenesis of CCCA. **Table 1** lists the most commonly reported associated findings with CCCA along with their level of evidence.

DERMATOSCOPY

Dermatoscopy serves as a noninvasive diagnostic tool to elucidate specific findings seen in CCCA and to select the best sites for obtaining biopsy specimens. In a retrospective study, a highly sensitive and specific finding of a peripilar gray/white halo located around the emergence of hair follicles

Table 1
Conditions reported in association with CCCA

Associated Condition	Type of Study	Participants	Results
Uterine leiomyomas (Source: Dina, Okoye, Aguh, 2018)[17]	Retrospective cohort study	Black women (N = 487,104) • 447 women with CCCA and 486, 657 race-, age-, and sex-matched controls	• Statistically significant ($P<.001$)
Diabetes mellitus type II (Source: Kyei, Bergfeld, Piliang, Summers, 2011)[8]	Population study	Black women (N = 326)	• Statistically significant ($P = .01$)
Bacterial scalp infections (Source: Kyei, Bergfeld, Piliang, Summers, 2011)[8]	Population study	Black women (N = 326)	• Statistically significant ($P = .045$)

Abbreviation: CCCA, central centrifugal cicatricial alopecia.

was observed in 94% of patients diagnosed with CCCA.[18] Other reported dermatoscopic findings include honeycomb pigmented rete ridges and hypomelanotic dermal papillae, hair shaft variability, perifollicular erythema, and/or broken hairs presenting as black dots.[19] Dermatoscopic sites yielding these findings represent the best areas for biopsy and further examination to aid in the diagnosis of CCCA.

HISTOPATHOLOGY

Histopathologic analysis is useful in the diagnosis of CCCA and specific features can help distinguish CCCA from other scarring alopecias. The histopathology of CCCA is usually summarized by the presence of premature desquamation of the inner root sheath (PDIRS) at the level of the deep dermis with varying degrees of perifollicular lymphocytic inflammation around the infundibulum and isthmus that leads to follicular destruction and replacement of hair shafts with fibrosis.[20] PDIRS is such a sensitive finding, that its histologic presence in a patient with hair breakage is highly suggestive of CCCA even in the absence of other histologic features. However, although PDIRS is a sensitive finding, it is important to remember that this finding is not specific, therefore the presence of other histologic features should be examined to rule out other pathologies. A retrospective study[21] systematically described common histopathologic features discovered via serial horizontal sections of 51 cases. These findings are summarized in **Table 2** with relative frequencies of each finding within the study population. Other histologic findings associated with CCCA include eccentric atrophy of the outer root sheath, concentric lamellar fibroplasia at the level of the upper isthmus and lower infundibulum,[22] and even the presence of hair granulomas.[20] A recent study using scanning electron microscopy also reported the presence of atypical hair shaft characteristics consistent with pili trianguli et canaliculi in a black patient with CCCA.[23]

CLINICAL PRESENTATION

CCCA typically begins as an area of decreased hair density or hair breakage notably at the vertex of the scalp and expands peripherally (**Fig. 1**). In early stages, patients may report scalp pruritus or tenderness. The hair loss can progress insidiously, delaying diagnosis and treatment especially in asymptomatic patients. Advanced cases reveal impressive hair loss evidenced by a smooth, shiny scalp with loss of follicular ostia (**Fig. 2**). Hair breakage also can be a sign of early or occult

Table 2
Histopathologic features and frequencies associated with CCCA

Histopathologic Finding	Frequency, %
Premature desquamation of the inner root sheath below level of the isthmus	96
Absent or only focally preserved sebaceous glands, with the remnants presenting as lobules surrounding vellus hair follicles described as a "hugging" pattern	94
Individual or clusters of follicles surrounded by perifollicular fibrosis with varying degrees of inflammatory infiltrate	89
Follicular miniaturization	81
Lamellar hyperkeratosis with parakeratosis within the hair canal	79
Naked hair shafts	68

Abbreviation: CCCA, central centrifugal cicatricial alopecia.
Data from Miteva M, Tosti A. Pathologic diagnosis of central centrifugal cicatricial alopecia on horizontal sections. *Am J Dermatopathol* 2014;36(11):859-867.

CCCA, as shown in **Fig. 3**. In one study, 5 (63%) of 8 biopsy specimens demonstrated histologic changes of CCCA in African American patients presenting with hair breakage localized to the vertex with or without scalp symptoms.[20] A patchy form of CCCA (**Fig. 4**) has recently been described,[24] with hair loss occurring in patches along the lateral and posterior scalp highlighting the clinical variability that can pose diagnostic difficulty.

PATIENT EVALUATION OVERVIEW

When evaluating a patient with suspected CCCA, a thorough history should be obtained from the patient. **Box 1** lists pertinent questions applicable to patients with suspected CCCA. Baseline photographs of the affected area(s) are important to evaluate the patient's condition at subsequent follow-up visits. A detailed scalp examination using adequate lighting and a dermatoscope is necessary. Dermoscopy is essential in identifying the optimal site for a biopsy and narrowing the differential diagnosis.[19] We recommend performing scalp biopsies to establish a confirmatory

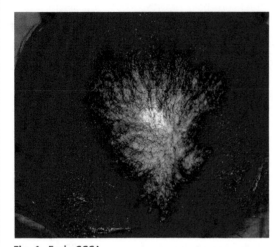

Fig. 1. Early CCCA.

diagnosis and to evaluate the extent of inflammation and/or scarring on histopathology. Two 4-mm punch biopsies, including both horizontal and vertical sectioning, should be obtained from the active border of the hair loss or symptomatic area.[25]

Table 3[2,26–28] provides a useful resource in differentiating the most common causes of central hair loss in African American women, which include CCCA, AGA, discoid lupus erythematosus (DLE), acquired trichorrhexis nodosa (TN), and tinea capitis. Other less common entities included in the differential diagnosis of CCCA include lichen planopilaris and folliculitis decalvans. The clinical pattern of alopecia in systemic lupus erythematosus has a more variable presentation as it has been reported to have both nonscarring (diffuse, patchy, or lupus hair pattern) and scarring forms

(as in DLE).[29] Symptoms of inflammatory-stage CCCA may include pruritus, tenderness, and a burning or altered sensation of the scalp. These clinical characteristics can help distinguish CCCA from the more common AGA, which is largely asymptomatic. In addition, clinical correlation with the use of dermoscopy and histologic evaluation can help establish the diagnosis. Because both CCCA and tinea capitis can present with pruritus, scaling, and hair breakage, a potassium hydroxide (KOH) preparation or fungal culture may be warranted to exclude the latter.

CCCA is unique compared with other forms of scarring hair loss in that fibrosis, as compared with inflammation, is often a striking clinical finding.[30] A central scalp alopecia photographic scale has been developed and validated to help correlate clinical information with the pattern and severity of central hair loss in African American women.[5] **Fig. 5** illustrates this scale in which pattern 0 is normal hair density and pattern 5 is hair loss over the entire top of the scalp. It is worth mentioning that some patients present with neither an anterior nor posterior presentation, but rather a central accentuation.

Dermoscopic findings of severe and mild CCCA are demonstrated in **Figs. 6** and **7**, respectively. This can be contrasted to the findings seen in dermoscopy of normal scalp (**Fig. 8**) and female pattern hair loss (**Fig. 9**).

TREATMENT
General Guidelines

The general goals in treating CCCA are aimed at addressing symptoms at the earliest presentation,

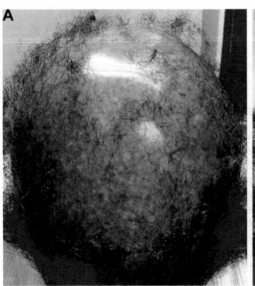

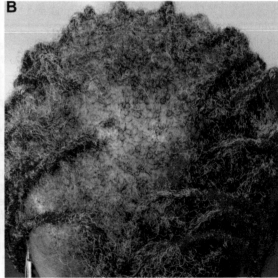

Fig. 2. (*A, B*) Late CCCA.

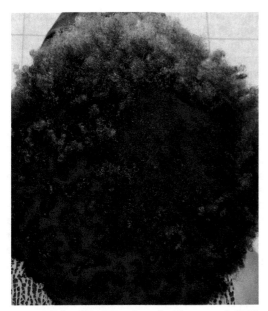

Fig. 3. Hair breakage as a sign of early or occult CCCA.

halting progression of disease, and establishing hair regrowth. These steps involve patient education, topical agents, systemic medications, and in some cases, procedural therapies. Discontinuation of hair grooming practices that promote fragility, tension, and trauma to the hair follicle is essential.[31] It is also important to acknowledge the psychological impact that patients with CCCA may experience. Many women often express concern that their hair will never grow back, which can negatively impact their self-esteem and interpersonal relationships. However, in recent years, protective and natural hairstyles have become increasingly more popular, which provide many patients the ability to treat their CCCA while selecting from a wide variety of alternative, safer hairstyles. Despite its initial description more than 50 years ago, large, randomized,

controlled trials on CCCA are lacking. For most patients with CCCA, combination therapy is often superior to monotherapy in demonstrating successful outcomes.[25] A proposed treatment algorithm is shown in **Fig. 10**.

Anti-inflammatory Phase

The first-line treatment for inflammatory-stage CCCA initially involves high-potency topical corticosteroids applied to the scalp once daily to 3 times a week. These are aimed to decrease the inflammation and alleviate patient symptoms. The vehicle formulation of the topical corticosteroid should be individualized to match the patient's desired hairstyling preference. For example, African American women with a natural hairstyle often prefer ointments, whereas women with braids may prefer foam, and solutions may be useful for women who primarily wear wigs. Once stabilization is observed, the topical corticosteroid can be transitioned to 3 nights weekly for maintenance.[32] A 14-week, open-label study[22] consisting of 30 adult women of African descent with clinical evidence of mild CCCA demonstrated substantial improvements in pruritus, pain, tenderness, erythema, and scaling with the use of daily application of clobetasol propionate 0.05% foam. In this study, scalp biopsies performed at week 12 in comparison with their baseline scalp biopsies revealed considerable improvements in severe inflammation and perifollicular edema.

Intralesional corticosteroids, most commonly intralesional triamcinolone acetonide (IL TAC) are used as an adjunct to topical corticosteroids in decreasing the inflammation. A commonly used dosing schedule consists of IL TAC 5 to 10 mg/mL performed every 4 to 6 weeks for approximately 3 to 6 months.[25,32] Additional IL TAC treatments should be repeated as necessary for symptom flare ups or clinical signs of inflammation. Injections should be performed along the

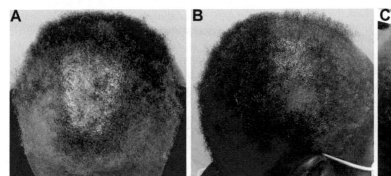
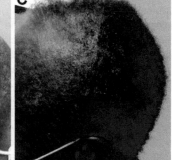

Fig. 4. (A–C) Patchy CCCA.

Box 1
Important questions to obtain when evaluating for central centrifugal cicatricial alopecia

When did you first notice your hair loss?

Have you experienced scalp burning, itching, or tenderness?

Is there a family history of similar hair loss?

How often do you wash your hair?

Do you use a blow dryer or air dry?

Do you chemically straighten ("relax") your hair? If so, how often?

Do you use a hot comb, flat iron, or curling iron?

Do you color your hair?

Do you style your own hair or have it professionally done by a hairstylist?

What treatment options have you previously tried to regrow your hair (including over-the-counter, prescription, and "natural" medicines)?

What hairstyles have you previously used and currently practice (eg, natural hairstyle, braids, weaves, wigs)?

Do you have any of the following medical conditions?

- Bacterial skin infections
- Diabetes mellitus type 2
- Fungal skin/scalp infections
- Hypertrophic scars or keloids
- Autoimmune disease (eg, lupus erythematosus)
- Sarcoidosis
- Seborrheic dermatitis (eg, dandruff)
- Thyroid disease
- Uterine fibroids

periphery of the areas of hair loss to prevent expansion of the inflammatory process.[25]

Many experts propose that the primary goal in treating patients with CCCA is halting disease progression at the earliest stage rather than regrowth of hair. This concept was demonstrated in a study[33] consisting of 15 African American women with biopsy-proven CCCA using photographs before and after treatment. The investigators found that despite no statistically significant difference in pretreatment versus posttreatment disease severity scores, topical steroids and intralesional steroids with or without minoxidil

and antidandruff shampoos halt disease progression.[33]

Oral antibiotics, most commonly doxycycline hyclate, are used for more moderate inflammatory symptoms or actively spreading disease. A dosing schedule of doxycycline hyclate 100 mg taken twice daily for 3 months is typically recommended. Once the process is stabilized, the oral antibiotic can be tapered down and the patient should continue their topical regimen with close clinical follow-up.[32] Minocycline is less commonly prescribed because of a higher rate of adverse events, including severe drug hypersensitivity reactions.[34,35] Additional off-label medical therapies, such as topical calcineurin inhibitors[36] and hydroxychloroquine,[37] have been used for CCCA. Recalcitrant cases of CCCA may be treated with mycophenolate mofetil, cyclosporine, or thalidomide.[19,32] In cases of active inflammation, short courses of oral corticosteroids can be used.[27]

Some African American women with CCCA have coexistent seborrheic dermatitis, which is often due to the differences in hair washing frequency. Patients with CCCA are often encouraged to cleanse their scalp at least every 1 to 2 weeks with an antifungal shampoo, such as ciclopirox 1% shampoo or ketoconazole 2% shampoo, which help to decrease the pruritus, inflammation, and scaling.[25] To combat the dryness associated with antidandruff shampoos, patients are encouraged to apply the medicated shampoo directly to the scalp, followed by a moisturizing shampoo and conditioner to the hair shafts.[38] In general, ketoconazole shampoo is prescribed less frequently for African American women because of the concern for increased hair fragility on the hair shafts.[39,40]

Regrowth Phase

Once anti-inflammatory therapies have improved the patient's symptoms over several months, a maintenance regimen aimed at preservation and regrowth of existing follicles should be established. Topical minoxidil (2% or 5% solution or 5% foam) is recommended for patients with CCCA to prolong the anagen phase of the hair follicles.[33] One study reported that 81% of cases of biopsy-proven CCCA demonstrated follicular miniaturization on horizontal sections, which supports the rationale for using minoxidil in the treatment of CCCA.[21] A maintenance program for CCCA often consists of a mid-potency topical corticosteroid 3 nights per week, topical minoxidil daily, an antiseborrheic shampoo every 1 to 2 weeks, and IL TAC as needed.[25] **Fig. 11**

Table 3
Common causes of central hair loss in African American women[2,26–28]

Type of Alopecia	Clinical Presentation	Dermoscopy	Histopathology
Androgenetic alopecia (AGA)	Male pattern: • Recession of the frontal hairline • Decreased hair density along the vertex, crown, frontal or bitemporal regions Female pattern: • Diffuse thinning • Gradual widening of the part	Hair shaft diameter variation of more than 20% hair shafts Peripilar halo (early) Predominance of single hair-bearing follicles Hypertrophy of sebaceous glands	Follicular miniaturization
Central centrifugal cicatricial alopecia (CCCA)	Early: • Erythema • Hair breakage • Hair thinning at the crown and/or vertex with symmetric expansion centrifugally • Irregular patchy alopecia at the central, lateral and posterior scalp • Follicular pustules • Scaling Late: • Shiny, smooth scalp • Loss of follicular ostia • Polytrichia • Dyspigmentation	Peripilar white-gray halo 1 or 2 hairs emerging together Peripilar erythema White patches of follicular scarring interrupting a honeycomb pigmented network Broken hairs/black dots Hair shaft variability	Varying degrees of perifollicular lymphohistiocytic inflammation Premature desquamation of the inner root sheath Concentric lamella fibroplasia
Discoid lupus erythematosus (DLE)	• Well-circumscribed round erythematous, infiltrative scaly plaques • Follicular plugging • Atrophy • Pigmentary changes • Scarring	Vacuolar interface change Superficial and deep perivascular and periadnexal lymphoplasmacytic infiltrate Variable amounts of deep dermal mucin Infundibular hyperkeratosis with ostial plugging Direct immunofluorescence may show immunoglobulin G and C3 along the dermoepidermal junction	Peripilar erythema and white scales Keratotic plug Thick arborizing vessels Scattered dark-brown discoloration Follicular red dots
Acquired trichorrhexis nodosa (TN)	• Dry, fragile, lusterless hair • Hair breakage • Characteristic "whitish spots" along the hair	Small white nodes at irregular intervals along hair shaft Fraying or breakage of the cortical fibers resembling "paintbrush fracture" or "broomstick" appearance	Cuticular cell disruption

(continued on next page)

Table 3 (continued)			
Type of Alopecia	Clinical Presentation	Dermoscopy	Histopathology
Tinea capitis	• Erythema • Pruritus • Pustules • Scaling	Comma hairs Broken hair shafts with scaling in "black dot" tinea Blotchy pigmentation	Dependent on causative organism (see below) Endothrix: fungal elements within the hair shaft (often *Trichophyton tonsurans*) Ectothrix: fungal elements coat the outside of the hair shaft (often *Microsporum* species)

demonstrates before and after photographs of a patients with CCCA who underwent medical therapy.

Procedural modalities for the treatment of CCCA include hair transplantation and platelet-rich plasma (PRP). In general, these methods should be reserved for patients with late-stage CCCA who have been well controlled on stable medical therapy for at least 9 to 12 months and demonstrate a lack of inflammation histologically.[41] Therefore, a scalp biopsy demonstrating absence of inflammation in the dermis should be documented before undergoing hair transplant surgery.[42] A case report of 2 African American female individuals with biopsy-proven CCCA demonstrated successful hair regrowth at both recipient sites following hair transplantation using the round punch grafting technique.[43] In this report, no postoperative scarring at the recipient or donor sites were noted in either patient. It is important to counsel patients on the potential need for multiple hair transplant sessions, possibility of disease recurrence, and proper maintenance therapy for stable control of CCCA.

PRP is defined as a plasma fraction of autologous blood that contains a greater concentration of platelets, typically threefold to sevenfold, relative to whole blood.[44] PRP relies on the activation of platelets that subsequently release a myriad of growth factors, such as PDGF, transforming growth factor beta (TGF-ß), vascular endothelial growth factor, and epidermal growth factor, which work to increase hair growth, stimulate angiogenesis, and promote hair-cell proliferation and regeneration.[42] In recent years, the use of PRP injections has become very popular in the treatment of AGA, but there are limited studies evaluating its efficacy in primary cicatricial alopecias. A recent case series of 2 patients with primary cicatricial alopecia highlighted successful treatment with PRP after 3 treatments spaced

4 weeks apart in an African American woman with biopsy-proven CCCA.[45] The investigators also found a reduction in the follicular density of treated areas within 6 months of stopping treatment, which supports the need for maintenance therapy with PRP.[46]

Although there is significant variability in PRP protocols, 1 study evaluating the efficacy of 2 different PRP regimens for AGA found that the benefits of PRP may be greater if first administered monthly as compared with every 3 months.[47] The precise mechanism for which PRP is effective in scarring alopecias such as CCCA is not completely understood; however, it is likely related to the host of growth factors that are upregulated and released on platelet activation. These include beta-catenin, which leads to differentiation of stem cells into hair follicle cells, MMP-1 and MMP-3, which degrade damaged extracellular matrix and promote synthesis of new collagen through increased production of procollagen type 1, and TGF-ß and TGF-ß1 which are anti-inflammatory and proangiogenic cytokines.[45,48] In the senior author's experience, the use of PRP is most advantageous in women who have concomitant CCCA and AGA. **Fig. 12** demonstrates before and after photographs of a patient with biopsy-proven concomitant CCCA and AGA treated with topical steroids, doxycycline, and 5 sessions of PRP within a 9-month timeframe.

New Developments

Two recent case reports of African American female individuals with advanced stage CCCA were shown to demonstrate visible hair regrowth with use of a compounded topical metformin 10% cream applied to the scalp daily after 4 to 6 months.[49] Scalp dryness and irritation were reported, which diminished with application of a topical emollient or moisturizer. Neither patient

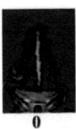

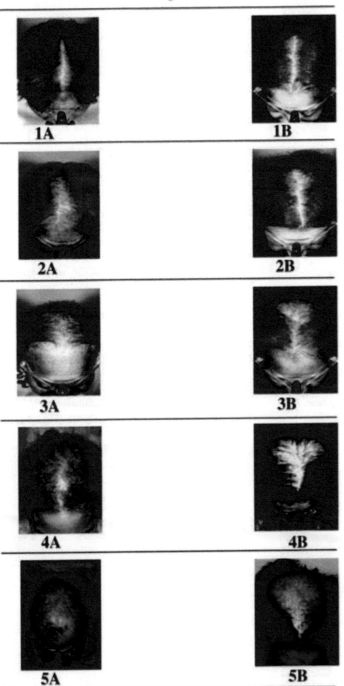

Fig. 5. Central scalp alopecia photographic scale in African American women. (*From* Olsen E, Callender V, Sperling L, et al. Central scalp alopecia photographic scale in African American women. Dermatol Ther 2008;21(4):264-7; with permission.)

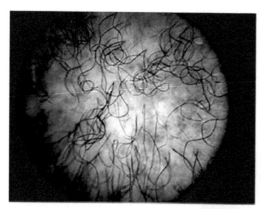

Fig. 6. Dermoscopy in CCCA. The presence of a peripilar white halo corresponds to the lamellar fibrosis surrounding the outer root sheath (ORS). Note the peripilar erythema, which indicates intense perifollicular inflammation.

experienced adverse systemic side effects. The investigators propose that metformin's beneficial role in CCCA may stem from its effect through activation of adenosine monophosphate-activated protein kinase, which plays an important role in mediating fibrosis.[49]

THE ROLE OF HAIR CARE PRACTICES

The differences in hair structure in patients of African ancestry compared with other ethnic backgrounds plays an important role when discussing treatments for CCCA. In its natural state, the African hair shaft tends to be elliptical or flattened in cross-section and spiral or tightly curled in its tertiary structure.[38] It is important to note that not all patients of African descent exhibit curly hair. African hair also exhibits more knots, broken hair shafts, and interlocking of hair shafts.[50] These

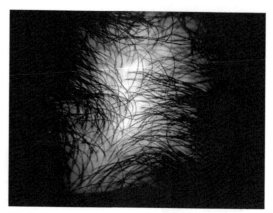

Fig. 8. Dermoscopy in normal scalp.

characteristics largely account for the weakness and increased fragility of the African hair follicle.[19] The incorporation of certain hair grooming practices can further increase the risk for hair breakage and trauma.

A retrospective comparative survey of 101 African American women reported a strong association between the use of both sewn-in hair weaving and cornrow or braided hairstyles with artificial hair extensions and CCCA ($P<.04$).[15] In this study, the patients with CCCA who reported these 3 hairstyles were more likely to report a history of hair damage with symptoms including scalp tenderness and uncomfortable pulling. Interestingly, in this same study, no correlation was found between the use of either hot combing or hair relaxers and the development of CCCA.[15]

This is important to keep in mind, as currently there is a movement in the African American community to wear hair in its naturally curly state (**Fig. 13**) or use protective styles (**Fig. 14**) as

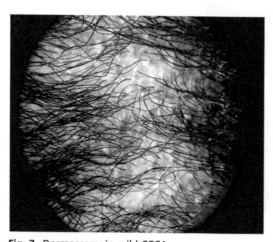

Fig. 7. Dermoscopy in mild CCCA.

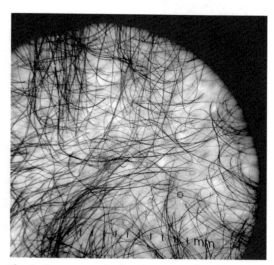

Fig. 9. Dermoscopy in female pattern hair loss.

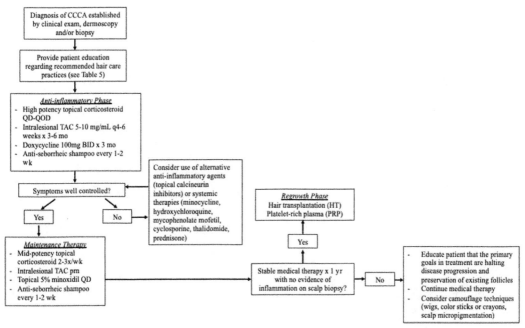

Fig. 10. Treatment algorithm in CCCA. BID, twice a day; prn, as needed; QD, once a day; QOD, every other day.

opposed to the use of chemical relaxers, straighteners, and hot combs, which can potentially damage the hair. With this shift comes new strategies to manage hair, with the principles largely based on (1) minimal hair manipulation by use of protective styles such as box braids and wigs, and (2) an emphasis on hydration by use of essential oils to retain moisture in the hair. These strategies are very popular on social media, under the notion that they prevent breakage and maintain the health of the hair. It will be interesting to see if this plays a role into the incidence of CCCA in the future for

those opting to maintain their hair in its natural state and for those transitioning from chemical processing.

Although recent literature demonstrates that CCCA has a multifactorial cause rather than hair care practices as the main culprit, it is critical that patients with CCCA are educated on the importance of discontinuation of potentially damaging hair grooming practices, which could further exacerbate their disease state. This includes encouraging patients to avoid chemical straightening, decreasing heat to the scalp, and

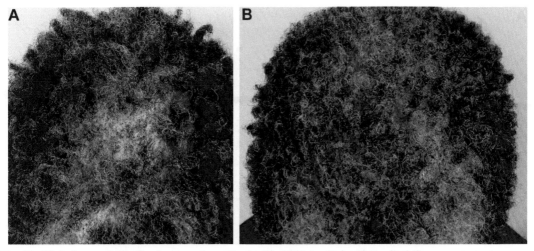

Fig. 11. (A) Before and (B) after images of a patient with CCCA treated with medical therapy.

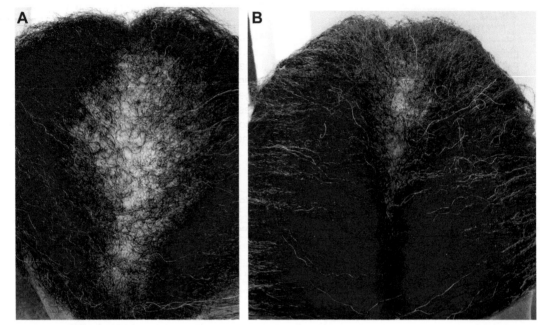

Fig. 12. (*A*) Before and (*B*) after the fifth session of PRP in a patient with biopsy-proven concomitant CCCA and AGA. Previous medical therapies included topical steroids and doxycycline. Photographs were taken approximately 9 months apart.

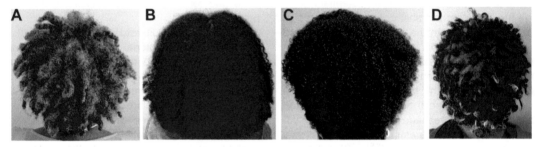

Fig. 13. (*A–D*) Female individuals with natural hair.

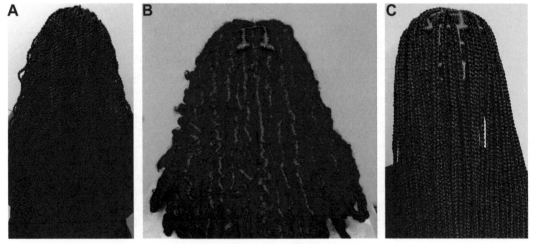

Fig. 14. (*A–C*) Protective styles: (*A*) twists, (*B*) faux dreadlocks, (*C*) box braids.

avoiding hairstyles that promote traction, such as tight braids and sewn-in or glued-in weaves.[37] Hardening gels and sprays also should be avoided. For patients with CCCA who continue to chemically straighten or "relax" the hair, it is important to advise them to seek professional care at a salon, apply a base (usually petrolatum equivalent) to the entire scalp before the relaxer, use a milder strength formulation, and decrease the frequency of relaxer touch-ups to every 8 to 10 weeks.[32] **Box 2** includes helpful hairstyling tips for women with CCCA. For patients with advanced, late-stage CCCA, camouflage techniques such as wigs, color sticks or crayons, and scalp micropigmentation are additional options. Although there is a lack of data documenting success of scalp micropigmentation (SMP) specifically for the treatment of CCCA, one study[51] of 43 Korean patients found micropigmentation to be a useful method for camouflaging pattern alopecia and scalp scars. Another study[52] reported moderate to great improvement after SMP with satisfactory scalp coverage in 30 patients with hair loss, including 3 patients with cicatricial alopecia, 3 patients with alopecia areata, and 24 patients with AGA.

CHALLENGES AND SOLUTIONS

Early CCCA can often be difficult to distinguish from the most common form of alopecia, which is AGA. Unfortunately, this can pose a major challenge and delay appropriate treatment. CCCA in men can present almost identical to AGA; however, the former usually presents at an earlier age, is symptomatic, and is restricted to the vertex, whereas the latter can have asymptomatic additional hair loss in the frontal or bi-temporal hairline or crown.[12] This highlights the importance in performing a scalp biopsy for confirmation. Typical findings of CCCA on histopathologic analysis include lamellar fibroplasia, PDIRS, and perifollicular inflammation.[12]

Because of the insidious progression of CCCA, many asymptomatic women have this condition years before presenting to a dermatologist. Because the process occurs primarily at the crown or vertex, some may be completely unaware of their hair loss until someone brings it to their attention. Because many women of African descent visit licensed cosmetologists for routine hair care, it is important to properly educate them on recognizing this condition to promote early diagnosis and treatment.[37] Therefore, hairstylists have a critical role in detecting the earliest visible signs of CCCA. As previously mentioned, it is important to keep in mind that early CCCA should be included in the differential diagnosis of hair breakage at the crown or vertex, even in asymptomatic patients without obvious signs of scarring.[20] A biopsy should be performed in these cases to diagnose the condition in its earliest stage, which optimizes the patient's chance for successful outcomes. A cross-sectional survey study of 38 women with biopsy-proven CCCA demonstrated that the duration of hair loss was found to be strongly positively associated with the degree of hair loss, which reflects the progressive nature of CCCA.[53] However, with early recognition and prompt intervention, medical therapies can help to arrest the natural progression of CCCA.

Some dermatologists may not be as familiar with hair grooming practices unique to patients of African descent, which leads to challenges in effectively communicating how to select alternative hairstyles that limit tension and traction on the hair follicle. A cross-sectional survey study[54] of women diagnosed with CCCA found that the top 3 factors most important to patients with CCCA when seeking medical care included the physician's experience with black hair and CCCA (50%), the patient's personal hairstyling practice (26%), and the physician's ethnicity (26%). Dermatologists who may feel less familiar with CCCA can increase their knowledge of ethnic hair care practices by establishing mentorships or preceptorships with African American dermatologists working in private practice or academic multicultural centers well trained in treating CCCA. Selection of the most aesthetically pleasing topical vehicle for patients with CCCA is also important, as this increases compliance and improves patient outcomes.

Box 2
Hair grooming practices recommended for patients with central centrifugal cicatricial alopecia

Consider natural hairstyles (eg, avoid chemical and thermal straightening)

Limit heat (eg, use of blow dryer, curling iron, straightening or flat iron) to every 1 to 2 weeks if possible

Decrease all traumatic hairstyling methods that increase the risk for traction alopecia (tight braids, weaves)

Use camouflage techniques to decrease color contrast in advanced stages

- Match hair color with scalp color
- Apply color-matched keratin hair building fibers
- Wigs
- Scalp micropigmentation

Table 4
Common challenges and solutions encountered in CCCA

Challenges	Solutions
Early CCCA can be indistinguishable from AGA	• The presence of scalp pruritus, tenderness, or hair breakage localized to the vertex is suggestive of CCCA • Dermoscopy can help identify features specific and sensitive for CCCA, such as white/gray peripilar follicular halo • Dermoscopy in AGA may show the following: hair shaft diameter variation of more than 20% hair shafts, peripilar halo (early), predominance of single hair-bearing follicles, or hypertrophy of sebaceous glands
Fibrosis is often the predominant clinical finding in CCCA, whereas scalp inflammation is often less apparent compared with other forms of scarring alopecia	• Dermoscopy can help can identify the earliest signs of scalp fibrosis by visualization of loss of follicular ostia
CCCA can be misdiagnosed as seborrheic dermatitis, tinea capitis, or "chemically-treated" hair	• Educate primary care physicians and hairstylists on the importance of early diagnosis and treatment to slow progression of scarring and permanent hair loss • In patients whose symptoms worsen with topical steroids, maintain a high index of suspicion for tinea capitis and perform a potassium hydroxide preparation or fungal culture • Hair breakage localized to the crown or vertex can be an early marker for CCCA and diagnostic workup should include dermoscopy and/or biopsy • The use of dermoscopy aids in distinguishing other causes of alopecia that may mimic CCCA
Lack of physician familiarity and knowledge of hair care practices unique to women of African descent can lead to communication barriers	• Encourage dermatologists in residency training, academics and private practice to seek alternative approaches to overcome barriers in understanding hair grooming practices unique to patients of African descent • Choose an aesthetically pleasing topical vehicle for patients with CCCA (eg, natural hair – ointment; weave – solution; braids – foam)
Hair transplantation into areas of scar tissue can result in possibly decreased graft survival rates	• Ensure patient has had stable medical therapy for at least 9–12 mo • Perform repeat scalp biopsy to confirm lack of inflammation histologically • Before a full hair transplant procedure, perform a test session • Use larger punch grafts and larger recipient sites to minimize risk of transection of curved hair follicles
CCCA can have a negative impact on quality of life	• Establish early diagnosis and initiate prompt treatment to halt the progression of scarring and maximize chance for regrowth • Offer psychological support • Encourage patients to join educational resources such as the Cicatricial Alopecia Research Foundation (https://www.carfintl.org/) or Skin of Color Society (https://skinofcolorsociety.org/)

Abbreviations: AGA, androgenetic alopecia; CCCA, central centrifugal cicatricial alopecia.

Hair transplantation should be performed in appropriately selected patients with CCCA due to certain technical challenges in treating this scarring alopecia as compared with forms of nonscarring alopecia. One major concern with transplanting healthy follicles into recipient scar tissue is decreased graft viability, which is thought to be due to limited vascular supply.[41] Because African hair is naturally tightly curled and spiral in nature, there is an increased risk of transection during hair transplant surgery.[42] Therefore, a "test graft session" should initially be performed with close observation over the next 3 to 6 months to evaluate graft survival and hair regrowth.[25] This can be achieved by harvesting 5 to 6 round, 4-mm-sized punch grafts from the healthy posterior donor area and transplanting them into 5 to 6 round, 3.5-mm-sized recipient sites in the area of scarring.[41]

Once the test session has confirmed successful hair regrowth in the recipient site, a full hair transplant procedure can be performed. Although the more popular follicular unit extraction method has been used in some cases of scarring alopecia,[55] the more traditional punch graft technique[56] has demonstrated success in women with CCCA.[43] The advantages of using larger punch grafts, as opposed to smaller follicular units, include a decreased risk of transection of tightly curled hair follicles, improved hair density, optimal scalp coverage, and enhancement of follicle survival.[41] In addition, the presence of curly African hair can also create an appearance of denser growth and greater volume.[25]

Finally, studies have shown that the psychological burden and quality of life is more greatly impacted in women with scarring alopecia compared with those with nonscarring alopecia.[57] Furthermore, the negative impact of alopecia on quality of life is often more profound in younger patients compared with older patients.[58] Anxiety, depression, and low self-esteem have also been reported in numerous studies evaluating the impact on quality of life in women with many different forms of alopecia.[59] Similar to previous observational studies, one pilot study found that CCCA is a contributor to self-esteem challenges.[54] **Table 4** summarizes a list of commonly encountered challenges and solutions in the diagnosis and management of CCCA.

SUMMARY

CCCA remains the leading cause of scarring alopecia in women of African descent. Although certain traumatic hairstyles play a contributory role, we now understand this is a much more complex disease process. Future research will hopefully identify the exact inheritance pattern of CCCA, other causal genes linked to CCCA, and systemic diseases that we should screen for in our patients diagnosed with CCCA. In addition, future clinical studies should explore possible therapeutic options that target fibroproliferative genes upregulated in CCCA. As our understanding of CCCA continues to unravel, we hope that future treatments will help optimize the chance of reversing what we previously thought to be a permanent, irreversible form of alopecia.

CLINICS CARE POINTS

- CCCA is the most common form of primary scarring alopecia in women of African descent.[41]

- At the molecular level, an autosomal dominant mode of inheritance,[13] mutations in protein *PADI3*,[14] and upregulation of critical fibroproliferative genes[16] have all been linked to patients with CCCA.

- CCCA often occurs in the absence of clinical signs of overt inflammation and instead fibrosis is often the predominant feature.[30]

- The presence of a white/gray peripilar follicular halo on dermoscopy is both sensitive and specific for CCCA and should be followed up with biopsy for confirmatory diagnosis,[18]

- Treatment of CCCA can be divided into 2 stages (anti-inflammatory phase and regrowth phase) and more published case-controlled studies are needed.

DISCLOSURE

The authors have no disclosures to report.

REFERENCES

1. LoPresti P, Papa CM, Kligman AM. Hot comb alopecia. Arch Dermatol 1968;98:234–8.
2. Sperling LC, Sau P. The follicular degeneration syndrome in black patients: 'hot comb alopecia' revisited and revised. Arch Dermatol 1992;128:68–74.
3. Nicholson AG, Harland CC, Bull RH, et al. Chemically induced cosmetic alopecia. Br J Dermatol 1993;128:537–41.
4. Olsen EA, Bergfeld WF, Cotsarelis G, et al. Summary of North American Hair Research Society (NAHRS)-sponsored work-shop on cicatricial alopecia, Duke

University Medical Center, February 10 and 11, 2001. J Am Acad Dermatol 2003;48(1):103–10.

5. Olsen E, Callender V, Sperling L, et al. Central scalp alopecia photographic scale in African American women. Dermatol Ther 2008;21(4):264–7.

6. Olsen EA, Callender VD, McMichael A, et al. Central hair loss in African American women: incidence and potential risk factors. J Am Acad Dermatol 2011;64: 245–52.

7. Callender VD, Onwudiwe O. Prevalence and etiology of central centrifugal cicatricial alopecia. Arch Dermatol 2011;147(8):972–4.

8. Kyei A, Bergfeld WF, Piliang M, et al. Medical and environmental risk factors for the development of central centrifugal cicatricial alopecia: a population study. Arch Dermatol 2011;147:909–14.

9. Khumalo NP, Jessop S, Gumedze F, et al. Hairdressing and the prevalence of scalp disease in African adults. Br J Dermatol 2007;157:981–8.

10. Eginli AN, Dlova NC, McMichael A. Central centrifugal cicatricial alopecia in children: a case series and review of the literature. Pediatr Dermatol 2017;34(2): 133–7.

11. Sperling LC, Skelton HG 3rd, Smith KJ, et al. Follicular degeneration syndrome in men. Arch Dermatol 1994;130(6):763–9.

12. Davis EC, Reid SD, Callender VD, et al. Differentiating central centrifugal cicatricial alopecia and androgenetic alopecia in african american men: report of three cases. J Clin Aesthet Dermatol 2012;5(6):37–40.

13. Dlova NC, Jordaan FH, Sarig O, et al. Autosomal dominant inheritance of central centrifugal cicatricial alopecia in black South Africans. J Am Acad Dermatol 2014;70(4):679–82.e1.

14. Malki L, Sarig O, Romano MT, et al. Variant PADI3 in central centrifugal cicatricial alopecia. N Engl J Med 2019;380(9):833–41.

15. Gathers RC, Jankowski M, Eide M, et al. Hair grooming practices and central centrifugal cicatricial alopecia. J Am Acad Dermatol 2009;60: 674–8.

16. Aguh C, Dina Y, Talbot CC Jr, et al. Fibroproliferative genes are preferentially expressed in central centrifugal cicatricial alopecia. J Am Acad Dermatol 2018; 79(5):904–12.e1.

17. Dina Y, Okoye G, Aguh C. Association of uterine leiomyomas with central centrifugal cicatricial alopecia. JAMA Dermatol 2018;154(2):213–4.

18. Miteva M, Tosti A. Dermatoscopic features of central centrifugal cicatricial alopecia. J Am Acad Dermatol 2014;71(3):443–9.

19. Herskovitz I, Miteva M. Central centrifugal cicatricial alopecia: challenges and solutions. Clin Cosmet Investig Dermatol 2016;9:175–81.

20. Callender VD, Wright DR, Davis EC, et al. Hair breakage as a presenting sign of early or occult central centrifugal cicatricial alopecia. Arch Dermatol 2012;148:1047–52.

21. Miteva M, Tosti A. Pathologic diagnosis of central centrifugal cicatricial alopecia on horizontal sections. Am J Dermatopathol 2014;36(11):859–67.

22. Callender V, Kazemi A, Young C, et al. Safety and efficacy of clobetasol propionate 0.05% emollient foam for the treatment of central centrifugal cicatricial alopecia. J Drugs Dermatol 2020;19(7):719–24.

23. Araoye EF, Thomas JAL, Roker LA, et al. Pili trianguli et canaliculi as a phenotypic subtype in patients with central centrifugal cicatricial alopecia: a scanning electron microscopy study. J Am Acad Dermatol 2020;83(4):1010–1.

24. Gomez-Zubiaur A, Saceda-Corralo D, Velez-Velázquez MD, et al. Central centrifugal cicatricial alopecia following a patchy pattern: a new form of clinical presentation and a challenging diagnosis for the dermatologist. Int J Trichology 2019;11(5): 216–8.

25. Callender VD, McMichael AJ, Cohen GF. Medical and surgical therapies for alopecias in black women. Dermatol Ther 2004;17(2):164–76.

26. Jain N, Doshi B, Khopkar U. Trichoscopy in alopecias: diagnosis simplified. Int J Trichology 2013; 5(4):170–8.

27. Bolduc C, Sperling LC, Shapiro J. Primary cicatricial alopecia: lymphocytic primary cicatricial alopecias, including chronic cutaneous lupus erythematosus, lichen planopilaris, frontal fibrosing alopecia, and Graham-Little syndrome. J Am Acad Dermatol 2016;75(6):1081–99.

28. Rodney IJ, Onwudiwe OC, Callender VD, et al. Hair and scalp disorders in ethnic populations. J Drugs Dermatol 2013;12(4):420–7.

29. Chanprapaph K, Udompanich S, Visessiri Y, et al. Nonscarring alopecia in systemic lupus erythematosus: a cross-sectional study with trichoscopic, histopathologic, and immunopathologic analyses. J Am Acad Dermatol 2019;81(6):1319–29.

30. Aguh C. Updates in our understanding of central centrifugal cicatricial alopecia. Cutis 2019;104(6): 316, 340.

31. Lawson CN, Hollinger J, Sethi S, et al. Updates in the understanding and treatments of skin & hair disorders in women of color. Int J Womens Dermatol 2015;1(2):59–75.

32. Gathers RC, Lim HW. Central centrifugal cicatricial alopecia: past, present, and future. J Am Acad Dermatol 2009;60(4):660–8.

33. Eginli A, Dothard E, Bagayoko CW, et al. A retrospective review of treatment results for patients with central centrifugal cicatricial alopecia. J Drugs Dermatol 2017;16(4):317–20.

34. Smith K, Leyden JJ. Safety of doxycycline and minocycline: a systematic review. Clin Ther 2005;27(9): 1329–42.

35. Tsuruta D, Someda Y, Sowa J, et al. Drug hypersensitivity syndrome caused by minocycline. J Cutan Med Surg 2006;10(3):131–5.

36. Semble AL, McMichael AJ. Hair loss in patients with skin of color. Semin Cutan Med Surg 2015;34(2):81–8.

37. Summers P, Kyei A, Bergfeld W. Central centrifugal cicatricial alopecia - an approach to diagnosis and management. Int J Dermatol 2011;50(12):1457–64.

38. McMichael AJ. Hair and scalp disorders in ethnic populations. Dermatol Clin 2003;21(4):629–44.

39. Elgash M, Dlova N, Ogunleye T, et al. Seborrheic dermatitis in skin of color: clinical considerations. J Drugs Dermatol 2019;18(1):24–7.

40. Taylor SC, Barbosa V, Burgess C, et al. Hair and scalp disorders in adult and pediatric patients with skin of color. Cutis 2017;100(1):31–5.

41. Dlova NC, Salkey KS, Callender VD, et al. Central centrifugal cicatricial alopecia: new insights and a call for action. J Investig Dermatol Symp Proc 2017;18:S54–6.

42. Okereke UR, Simmons A, Callender VD. Current and emerging treatment strategies for hair loss in women of color. Int J Womens Dermatol 2019;5(1):37–45.

43. Callender VD, Lawson CN, Onwudiwe OC. Hair transplantation in the surgical treatment of central centrifugal cicatricial alopecia. Dermatol Surg 2014;40(10):1125–31.

44. Hesseler MJ, Shyam N. Platelet-rich plasma and its utility in medical dermatology: a systematic review. J Am Acad Dermatol 2019;81(3):834–46.

45. Dina Y, Aguh C. Use of platelet-rich plasma in cicatricial alopecia. Dermatol Surg 2019;45(7):979–81.

46. Finney R. Commentary on use of platelet-rich plasma in cicatricial alopecia. Dermatol Surg 2019; 45(7):982–3.

47. Hausauer AK, Jones DH. Evaluating the efficacy of different platelet-rich plasma regimens for management of androgenetic alopecia: a single-center, blinded, randomized clinical trial. Dermatol Surg 2018;44(9):1191–200.

48. Arshdeep, Kumaran MS. Platelet-rich plasma in dermatology: boon or a bane? Indian J Dermatol Venereol Leprol 2014;80(1):5–14.

49. Araoye EF, Thomas JAL, Aguh C. Hair regrowth in 2 patients with recalcitrant central centrifugal cicatricial alopecia after use of topical metformin. JAAD Case Rep 2020;6(2):106–8.

50. Khumalo NP, Doe PT, Dawber RP, et al. What is normal black African hair? A light and scanning electron-microscopic study. J Am Acad Dermatol 2000;43(5 Pt 1):814–20.

51. Park JH, Moh JS, Lee SY, et al. Micropigmentation: camouflaging scalp alopecia and scars in Korean patients. Aesthetic Plast Surg 2014;38(1):199–204.

52. Dhurat RS, Shanshanwal SJS, Dandale AL. Standardization of SMP procedure and its impact on outcome. J Cutan Aesthet Surg 2017;10(3):145–9.

53. Suchonwanit P, Hector CE, Bin Saif GA, et al. Factors affecting the severity of central centrifugal cicatricial alopecia. Int J Dermatol 2016;55(6):e338–43.

54. Akintilo L, Hahn EA, Yu JMA, et al. Health care barriers and quality of life in central centrifugal cicatricial alopecia patients. Cutis 2018;102(6):427–32.

55. Zhu DC, Liu PH, Fan ZX, et al. Extensive scarring alopecia treated through a single dense-packing follicular unit extraction megasession. Dermatol Surg 2021;47(1):e15–20.

56. Orentreich N. Autografts in alopecias and other selected dermatological conditions. Ann N Y Acad Sci 1959;83:463–79.

57. Katoulis AC, Christodoulou C, Liakou AI, et al. Quality of life and psychosocial impact of scarring and non-scarring alopecia in women. J Dtsch Dermatol Ges 2015;13(2):137–42.

58. Dlova NC, Fabbrocini G, Lauro C, et al. Quality of life in South African Black women with alopecia: a pilot study. Int J Dermatol 2016;55(8):875–81.

59. Davis DS, Callender VD. Review of quality of life studies in women with alopecia. Int J Womens Dermatol 2018;4(1):18–22.

Alopecia Areata
New Treatment Options Including Janus Kinase Inhibitors

Caiwei Zheng, BA[a], Antonella Tosti, MD[b],*

KEYWORDS

- Tofacitinib • Ruxolitinib • Baricitinib • Abatacept • Platelet-rich plasma

KEY POINTS

- Alopecia areata is a disease, and not a cosmetic problem.
- Drugs that target the JAK-STAT pathway are effective in inducing regrowth in a high percentage of patients.
- Numerous JAK inhibitors are undergoing clinical trials worldwide.
- Although effective, JAK inhibitors are a treatment, not a cure.

OVERVIEW

Alopecia areata (AA) is a chronic, relapsing, autoimmune disorder characterized by patchy non-scaring hair loss. There is significant variation in the clinical presentation of AA, but patients most commonly present with smooth, circular, well-demarcated patches of complete hair loss that occur over weeks. AA can affect patients of all age groups, sexes, and ethnicities, and is reported to affect approximately 0.1% to 0.2% of the general population.[1,2] The disease is uncommon in children younger than the age of 3, but overall affects a young population, with up to 66% of patients less than 30 years of age and only 20% older than age 40.[3,4] Patients with AA are also reported to have increased overall risk (16%) of concomitant autoimmune disorders, including systemic lupus erythematosus, vitiligo, and autoimmune thyroid disease.[5,6]

Pathogenesis

Hair follicles are unique as the only organ to experience lifelong cycling transformation.[7,8] Normally, the cycle involves a period of active growth (anagen), when pigmentation and hair shaft production occurs; a short, apoptotic involution phase (catagen); and a resting phase (telogen).[7,8] Hair follicles in the anagen stage are found to experience a downregulation of major histocompatibility class (MHC) I and II along with local production of immunosuppressive agents (eg, α-melanocyte-stimulating hormone, transforming growth factor-$\beta1$ and -$\beta2$), a milieu of features that confers an immune advantage by decreasing the likelihood of autoimmune attack on intrafollicular autoantigens.[9–11] Decrease in MHC I expression effectively reduces the chance of autoantigen recognition by CD8+ T cells.[9–11] Although lack of MHC class I makes the hair follicle more prone to natural killer (NK) cell attack, concomitant downregulation of NK cell receptor ligands and production of immunosuppressive factors, such as transforming growth factor-$\beta1$ and -$\beta2$, melanocyte-stimulating hormone, and macrophage migration inhibitory factor, protect against NK cell attack.[12] Together, these protective features are referred to as the immune privilege (IP).

[a] University of Miami Miller School of Medicine, 1150 Northwest 14th Street, Miami, FL 33136, USA; [b] Dr. Phillip Frost Department of Dermatology and Cutaneous Surgery, University of Miami Miller School of Medicine, 1150 Northwest 14th Street, Miami, FL 33136, USA
* Corresponding author.
E-mail address: atosti@med.miami.edu

Dermatol Clin 39 (2021) 407–415
https://doi.org/10.1016/j.det.2021.03.005
0733-8635/21/© 2021 Elsevier Inc. All rights reserved.

Although the pathogenesis of AA is not yet completely elucidated, loss of IP in anagen stage hair follicles is widely accepted to play a key role. This is supported by histologic examination of AA lesions, which characteristically show perifollicular T-lymphocyte infiltration and premature transition from anagen to the nonproliferative catagen and telogen phases. The cause of the loss is believed to be multifactorial, and genetic predisposition and environmental triggers, such as infectious pathogens, has been suggested. One theory postulated that patients with AA may have abnormal $CD8^+$ T-cell response, and that infection with Epstein-Barr virus in a different organ may trigger clonal expansion of autoreactive T cells, leading to infiltration of hair follicles.[13] Detection of cytomegalovirus DNA in scalp biopsies of patients with AA has also been reported, although this hypothesis is less supported. Regardless of the cause of the loss, restoration of IP is currently considered key to AA therapy.[14]

INVESTIGATIONAL TREATMENT

Although many treatment modalities have been proposed, there is currently no preventive or curative treatment of AA. Traditional therapy includes topical and systemic steroids, methotrexate, retinoids, topical immunotherapy (eg, squaric acid dibutylester, diphencyprone), hydroxychloroquine, minoxidil, and anthralin, but all are off-the-label use and yield varying, limited results. New treatment options are being actively developed and progress has been made over recent years. Treatment options currently under active investigation include various Janus kinase (JAK) inhibitors, interleukin (IL)-2 and -17, phenol, abatacept, and platelet-rich plasma (PRP), all of which are detailed in this article.

Janus Kinase Inhibitors

The JAK-signal transducer and activator of transcription (JAK-STAT) pathway is an intracellular signaling pathway at which numerous proinflammatory pathways converge. The pathway involves the JAK family of four kinases (JAK1, JAK2, JAK3, and tyrosine kinase 2 [TYK2]), which are located on the intracellular domains of the type I and II cytokine receptors to transduce ligand-binding signals when certain cytokines bind their receptors.[15,16] This activates binding and phosphorylation of the STAT family of DNA-binding proteins and leads to a cascade of downstream signaling that mediates cell proliferation, differentiation, migration, and apoptosis.[15,16] Several cytokines that depend on JAK signaling have been identified to be involved in AA, including IL-2, IL-7, IL-15, IL-

21, and interferon-γ, making JAK inhibitors an attractive therapeutic target (**Fig. 1**).

In 2014, a study by Xing and colleagues[17] presented evidence that AA is caused by $CD8^+NKG2D^+$ T cells via an IL-15-mediated positive feedback loop with follicular epithelial cells. The study used a mouse model using C3H/HeJ mice, a strain that has been found to develop AA that is considerably similar to human AA and demonstrated that antibody-mediated blockade of interferon-γ, IL-2, or IL-15 receptor β using ruxolitinib (JAK 1 and 2 inhibitor) and tofacitinib (JAK1 and 3 inhibitor) was able to prevent disease development and lead to a reduction of the accumulation of $CD8^+NKG2D^+$ T cells.[17] The study also included a clinical trial of three human patients with moderate/severe AA and became one of the first studies to suggest oral ruxolitinib, 20 mg, as an effective therapeutic agents to reverse established AA.[17] Since then, Mackay-Wiggan and coworkers,[18] Vandiver and colleagues,[19] and Liu and King[20] have all published clinical trials that offered evidence of ruxolitinib's utility in AA reversal citing good tolerability for up to 31 months of use. However, the effects of ruxolitinib have been reported to lack durability after discontinuation of treatment. For example, a third of the patients in the Mackay-Wiggan and coworkers[18] study were reported to have shedding starting 3 weeks after ruxolitinib discontinuation and had significant hair loss by Week 12, although not severe enough to revert to baseline levels.[18] The other two-thirds has also experienced increased shedding. As of October 2020, there are three ongoing clinical trials for ruxolitinib in progress and additional phase 2 trials of the investigational JAK1/2 inhibitor CTP-543, a deuterium-modified form of ruxolitinib, are also being conducted.

Tofacitinib citrate, a JAK1/3 inhibitor, is the most documented in literature for treatment of AA. In 2016, one large two-center open label clinical trial reported that of the 66 patients treated with twice-daily oral 5 mg tofacitinib, 32% experienced at least 50% improvement in Severity of Alopecia Tool (SALT) score.[21] However, of the 20 patients who consented for follow-up, disease relapse occurred in all 20 patients 8.5 weeks after drug cessation.[21] Adverse events included mild infections in 25.8% of patients, most commonly upper respiratory tract infections (16.7%), and headaches (7.6%). Later in 2017, a large (n = 90) cases series by Liu and colleagues[22] reported that 77% of patients responded to therapy after tofacitinib treatment with 58% of patients achieving greater than 50% change in SALT score after 4 to 18 months of treatment. Relapse information was not available in this study. More recently in 2019,

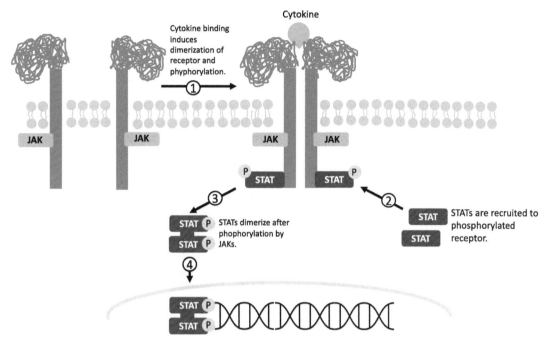

Cytokine

Cytokine binding induces dimerization of receptor and phyphorylation.

①

JAK   JAK   JAK   JAK

P STAT   STAT P

③ STAT P   STATs dimerize after phophorylation by STAT P   JAKs.

② STAT   STATs are recruited to phosphorylated STAT   receptor.

④ STAT P   STAT P

Dimerized STATs translocates to nucleus to activate gene trascription.

Fig. 1. JAK-STAT pathway and JAK inhibitors.

Almutairi and colleagues[23] published a randomized controlled clinical trial of 75 patients with severe AA treated with ruxolitinib and tofacitinib that reported a mean change in SALT score of 93.8 ± 3.25 in the ruxolitinib group and 95.2 ± 2.69 in the tofacitinib group, a substantial result. Unfortunately, two-thirds of the patients also experienced relapse by 3-month follow-up.[23]

Tofacitinib has also been used in adolescents and children with promising results reported in multiple studies. One study reported that in a retrospective cohort study of 13 adolescent patients of age 12 to 17, tofacitinib use at 5 mg twice daily dosing yielded a median SALT score improvement of 93% from baseline.[22] This was supported by another study that treated eight adolescents aged 12 to 19 with tofacitinib (5 mg twice a day) for a range of 5 to 18 months, yielding greater than 50% regrowth in scalp hair in all patients by 5 months.[24] As for pediatric patients, Craiglow and King[25] reported success treating four pediatric patients 8 to 10 years old with oral tofacitinib (5 mg twice a day) for a range of 6 to 15 months, with three of the four patients showing significant regrowth, and two of which showed complete regrowth by 6 months. In addition, baricitinib, a JAK 1 and 2 inhibitor, is another drug that has been used to treat AA. It is structurally similar to ruxolitinib but is unique in its ability to be metabolized independently of the cytochrome P-450 system and in that it is excreted renally. There is

much less information on baricitinib's use in AA but two recent case reports have reported significant hair regrowth with its use.[26,27] A large clinical trial comparing different doses of baricitinib in moderate severe AA is currently ongoing. A newer generation of JAK inhibitors that are more selective in their inhibition is also available. These selective JAK inhibitors are developed with the goal to more precisely induce inhibition of pathway components and reduce unwanted adverse effects. A list of the most well-known JAK inhibitors developed to date is available in **Table 1**, along with a comprehensive list of ongoing clinical trials exploring JAK inhibitor use in AA (**Table 2**).

Lastly, natural JAK inhibitors, such as curcumin (diferuloylmethane), the active phytochemical of turmeric, have been reported to have modulatory effects on JAK/STAT signaling.[18] Curcumin is a yellow pigment from the rhizomes of Curecuma longa and belongs to the family of polyphenols. A 2016 study by Zhao and colleagues[28] found that curcumin was able to attenuate trinitrobenzene sulfonic acid–induced experimental colitis in mice, hence alluding to its effect as a JAK inhibitor. However, there has yet to be clinical trials studying its use in alopecia.

Topical Treatment of Alopecia Areata

Topical treatments of AA exist, although results have not been consistent. For instance, topical

Table 1
JAK inhibitors by class

Class	Mechanism of Action	Drug Name
Nonselective	JAK1/2 inhibitor	Ruxolitinib[a] Baricitinib[a] CTP-543[a] Jaktinib
	JAK1/3 inhibitor	Tofacitinib[a] ATI-50002
	JAK1/TYK2 inhibitor	PF-06700841[a] SAR-20347
	Pan JAK inhibitor	Peficitinib Oclacitinib
Selective	JAK1 selective inhibitors	Filgotinib Upadacitinib Solcitinib PF-04965842 SHR0302
	JAK3 selective inhibitors	Decernotinib PF-06651600[a]
	TYK2 selective inhibitors	PF-06700841 BMS-986165 NDI-031232 NDI-031407
Natural JAK inhibitors	Curcumin (turmeric)	

[a] Has proven to be successful in treating AA.

2% tofacitinib has been reported to be effectively used in 11 patients age 4 to 16, yielding an average change of 32.3% in SALT score.[29] However, results were not long lasting and some saw loss of regrowth 9 to 12 months after starting therapy.[29] Topical ruxolitinib creams in 1% and 2% formulations have also been reported to yield regrowth of hair, particularly in lashes and scalp in patients with alopecia universalis. Bayart and colleagues[30] reported 75% regrowth of upper lashes in a 4-year-old pediatric patient treated with 2% ruxolitinib (twice a day for 3 months) and 95% of scalp hair in a 17-year-old patient treated with 1% ruxolitinib (twice a day for 18 months). Additionally, in a placebo-controlled, double-blind phase II and III clinical trial by Bokhari and Sinclair,[31] it was found that of 16 patients with AA, six demonstrated partial hair regrowth when treated with 2% tofacitinib twice a day and five demonstrated partial hair regrowth when treated with 1% ruxolitinib twice a day. No growth was observed in the placebo group. Of these patients with regrowth, some had maintained growth for up to 14 weeks later but some experienced relapse after 12 weeks.[31] However, there also exist case reports and clinical trials that report inconsistent or no induction of hair growth with topical ruxolitinib or tofacitinib cream.[31,32]

Abatacept

Up until 2010, the genetic basis of AA was largely unexplored. In 2010, a large genome-wide association study was conducted sampling 1050 cases and 3278 control subjects.[8] The study identified 139 single-nucleotide polymorphisms that are found to be significantly associated with AA and found associations with multiple genes that control key effectors of autoimmune disease, including: regulatory T cells, cytotoxic T-lymphocyte-associated antigen 4 (CTLA4), IL-2/IL-21, IL-2 receptor A (IL-2RA; CD25) and Eos or Ikaros family zinc finger 4 (IKZF4), and the HLA region.[8] The discovery that there is strong genetic susceptibility at the CTLA4 locus implicated that abatacept, a CTLA4-immunoglobulin costimulation modulator known to attenuate activation of T cells, may be a promising target for therapy.[33]

To date, only one clinical trial investigating the efficacy of abatacept in AA treatment has been published (Clinical trial identifier: NCT02018042). This is an open-label, single-arm clinical trial that treated 15 patients with moderate to severe AA, Alopecia totalis (AT), or Alopecia universalis (AU) using abatacept (subcutaneous injection at 125 mg daily) for 24 weeks.[33] Of the study participant, one participant demonstrated significant hair regrowth of greater than 50% increase from baseline at 18 weeks, and durable, complete regrowth by Week 36.[33] Four of the other participants showed intermediate clinical response with 15% to 25% hair regrowth at Week 24, four more participants showed 3% to 10% regrowth, and four more showed no response.[33] One patient demonstrated hair regrowth in the eyebrows but not scalp, and one was unable to complete the study. These results suggested that abatacept is a safe and effective alternative treatment of AA and may be particularly useful as a part of a combination therapy. Nonetheless, literature support for abatacept is still largely limited.

Platelet-Rich Plasma

PRP, also known as autologous conditioned plasma, is therapy using an injection of one's own platelet concentrate to accelerate cell proliferation and wound healing. Preparation of PRP involves collection of the patient's own whole blood, then centrifuging it to remove red blood cells, leaving a fraction with concentrated platelets and a variety of platelet-derived growth factors that is, on average, three to five times more concentrated

Table 2
Current status of clinical trials of JAK inhibitors for AA treatment listed on clinicaltrials.gov (October 2020)

Title of Trial Listing	Identifier	Molecule	Status	Location	Study Type	AA Type	Start Date
Effectiveness and Safety of Tofacitinib in Patients With Extensive and Recalcitrant Alopecia Areata	NCT03800979	Tofacitinib	Active, not recruiting	Bangkok, Thailand	Phase 4 cohort study with 19 participants	AA	January 12, 2019
Tofacitinib for Immune Skin Conditions in Down Syndrome	NCT04246372	Tofacitinib	Recruiting	Colorado, United States	Phase 2 open-label study with 46 participants	AA	October, 2020
PF-06651600 for the Treatment of Alopecia Areata	NCT03732807	PF-06651600	Active, not recruiting	Multicenter, United States	Phase 2b, 3 double-blind, placebo-controlled RCT with 718 participants	AA	December 3, 2018
Long-Term PF-06651600 for the Treatment of Alopecia Areata	NCT04006457	PF-06651600	Recruiting	Multicenter, United States	Phase 3 open-label study with 960 participants	AA	July 18, 2019
Placebo-Controlled Safety Study of Ritlecitinib (PF-06651600) in Adults with Alopecia areata	NCT04517864	PF-06651600	Recruiting	Multicenter, United States	Phase 2a double-blind, placebo-controlled RCT with 60 participants	AA	September 15, 2020
A Phase II Study in Patients with Alopecia Areata	NCT04346316	SHR0302	Recruiting	Multicenter, United States	Phase 2 double-blind, placebo-controlled RCT with 80 participants	AA	May 13, 2020
Jaktinib Dihydrochloride Monohydrate in Severe Alopecia Areata	NCT04034134	Jaktinib	Recruiting	Multicenter, China	Phase 2 RCT with 104 participants	AA	November 18, 2019
A Study With Jaktinib Hydrochloride Cream Applied Topically to Subjects With Alopecia Areata	NCT04445363	Jaktinib	Recruiting	Hunan, China	Phase 1, 2 RCT with 120 participants	AA	June 3, 2020

(continued on next page)

Table 2
(continued)

Title of Trial Listing	Identifier	Molecule	Status	Location	Study Type	AA Type	Start Date
Extension Study to Evaluate Safety and Efficacy of CTP-543 in Adults With Alopecia Areata	NCT03898479	CTP-543	Active, not recruiting	Multicenter, United States	Phase 2 open label study with 142 participants	AA	April 4, 2019
A Phase 3 Study to Evaluate the Efficacy and Safety of CTP-543 in Adult Patients With Moderate to Severe Alopecia Areata	NCT04518995	CTP-543	Active, not recruiting	Multicenter, United States	Phase 3 double-blind, placebo-controlled RCT with 700 participants	AA	October 2020
A Study of Baricitinib (LY3009104) in Participants With Severe or Very Severe Alopecia Areata	NCT03570749	Baricitinib	Active, not recruiting	Multicenter	Phase 2, 3 double-blind, placebo-controlled RCT with 725 participants	AA	September 24, 2018
A Study of Baricitinib (LY3009104) in Adults With Severe or Very Severe Alopecia Areata	NCT03899259	Baricitinib	Active, not recruiting	Multicenter	Phase 3 double-blind, placebo-controlled RCT with 476 participants	AA	July 8, 2019

Abbreviation: RCT, randomized controlled trial.

than whole blood.[34] PRP therapy is most established in orthopedics and dentistry to expedite healing of tissue damage but recent studies have reported that it can promote hair growth in vitro and in vivo.[35,36] In vitro, PRP is thought to increase the proliferation of dermal papilla cells, and stimulate extracellular signal-regulated kinase (ERK) and protein kinase B (Akt) signaling.[35] It was also reported to stimulate fibroblast growth factor-7 and beta-catenin, both of which are known hair follicle stimulators.[35] In vivo, Uebel and colleagues[36] demonstrated that hair grafts stored in PRP had enhanced graft survival, superior hair density, and enhanced growth of transplanted follicular units. In addition, PRP is reported to have anti-inflammatory effects, such as significant monocyte chemotactic protein-1 suppression, which also suggests efficacy against inflammatory dermatosis.[37] The exact mechanism PRP has on hair follicles is not yet elucidated.

Platelet-rich plasma as monotherapy

Trink and colleagues[34] first evaluated activated PRP use in AA in 2013. The team conducted a randomized, double-blind, split-scalp clinical trial involving 45 patients with chronic, relapsing AA (at least 2 years in duration) and compared PRP's efficacy with standard treatment of triamcinolone (TrA), 25 mg/mL, and a placebo treatment of distilled water.[34] Patients received monthly injections of either experimental treatment or control treatment over a period of 3 consecutive months. Results showed that patients treated with PRP had significantly increased hair regrowth compared with those treated with TrA and a higher percentage (60% vs 27%) achieved complete remission at 12 months.[34] This first established PRP as a potential safe and efficient alternative to standard AA treatment.

Activated PRP efficacy was further assessed by Shumez and colleagues[38] and El Taieb and colleagues,[39] who compared it with a higher dose of TrA (10 mg/mL) and topical 5% minoxidil, respectively. In the Shumez and colleagues' study,[38] only patients with mild AA (patients with <25% scalp or facial alopecia) were recruited, and the study treated 26 patients with PRP (vs 48 patients with TrA) once every 3 weeks for three sessions. Compared with high-dose TrA, PRP demonstrated earlier clinical response but results were not statistically significant, a discrepancy possibly caused by small sample size and limited room for improvement in mild AA cases.[38] In the study comparing PRP with 5% minoxidil, 90 subjects were treated monthly for 3 months, after which minoxidil and PRP showed significant hair growth compared with the placebo. However, there were no significant differences in results between the two groups, although the PRP group had an earlier clinical response and significantly greater reduction in vellus and dystrophic hairs.[39] More recently in 2019, Albalat and Ebrahim[40] conducted a double-blind randomized controlled trial with 80 patients comparing PRP efficacy with that of intralesional steroids and similarly found no significant difference in treatment results between the two groups, although significant hair regrowth and decrease in dystrophic hair was further confirmed.

Platelet-rich plasma as combined therapy

PRPs use as a part of combination therapy with other anti–hair loss agents has also been evaluated, but studies are limited in number and sample size. Results also mainly demonstrated improved clinical response with regards to hair shaft diameter rather than number. For instance, although PRP combined with 5% minoxidil topical solution and 1-mg oral finasteride is found to have a cumulative effect on dermal papilla cells and yielded superior hair count and anagen/telogen ratio compared with PRP alone in patients with androgenic alopecia, such effects have not been reported for patients with AA. For AA, the only report is from a case report published by Mubki[41] in 2016 that reported that combination therapy with PRP and intralesional TrA yielded only 4% higher hair regrowth by number of regrowth of terminal hairs compared with TrA alone (16% vs 12%) but showed a 39% larger hair fiber diameter.

Dupilumab

Of note, dupilumab (Dupixent), a human monoclonal antibody that acts as a dual IL-4 and IL-13 inhibitor that recently became available for treatment of atopic dermatitis (AD), has been found to yield significant improvement of AA in several case reports.[42–44] Patients reported in these case reports ranged from age 13 to 44 and all have coexisting AD, for which dupilumab was indicated. In one of these cases, a 13-year-old patient with a history of AD since age 7 and alopecia totalis since age 2 showed vellus hair growth on the scalp within 6 weeks of treatment with dupilumab (300-mg subcutaneous injection every other week), and considerable terminal hair growth by 11 months follow-up.[44] Shedding was noted when dupilumab was temporarily stopped during the treatment period. In another case, a 44-year-old man with a history of AD since childhood and an 8-year history of AA was treated with dupilumab (600-mg subcutaneous injection followed by 300 mg every 2 weeks), and saw a decrease in SALT score at the scalp from 61.6 to 8 in 3 months.[43] Although the pathogenesis of AA is incompletely understood, the efficacy seen in these cases is speculated to be caused by shared immune characteristics between AD and AA, although some suspect it may be an indirect effect from decreased inflammation from AD recovery.

SUMMARY AND FUTURE DIRECTIONS

Although there is not yet a safe, effective, curative treatment of AA, several agents targeting the various pathways implicated in AA pathogenesis have proved to be promising options within the past decade. Of these investigative treatment options, JAK inhibitors are the most supported by clinical trials and literature to date, although some drugs have been found to have limited durability in clinical response. There remains the need to determine a validated dosage for its use in AA treatment and the vehicles used for topical formulations has room for improvement in terms of effective skin penetration and limiting systemic absorption. Further studies are also needed to determine long-term safety of JAK inhibitor use. With the development of more selective JAK inhibitors, and a dozen new drugs in clinical trial, there is hope that JAK inhibitors can be added to the armamentarium of AA treatment in the near future.

CLINICS CARE POINTS

- Oral ruxolitinib 20 mg day has been reported to be an effective therapeutic agent to reverse established AA, but the effects lack durability after discontinuation of treatment.
- Oral tofacitinib 10 mg day has been shown to induce hair regrowth in moderate to severe alopecia areata, but relapse rate is high after discontinuation of treatment Several other oral JAK inhibitors are currently undergoing clinical trials including baricitinib and ritlecitinib.
- Topical JAK inhibitors such as 2% tofacitinib, 2% ruxolitinib and 1% ruxolitinib can be considered for eyebrows, eyelashes and beard area.

DISCLOSURE

Dr A. Tosti is consultant for DS Laboratories, Monat Global, Almirall, Tirthy Madison, Eli Lilly, Leo Pharmaceuticals, Bristol Myers Squibb, and P&G.

REFERENCES

1. John KKG, Brockschmidt FF, Redler S, et al. Genetic variants in CTLA4 are strongly associated with alopecia areata. J Invest Dermatol 2011;131:1169–72.

2. Höglund P, Brodin P. Current perspectives of natural killer cell education by MHC class I molecules. Nat Rev Immunol 2010;10(10):724–34.

3. Gilhar A, Etzioni A, Paus R. Alopecia areata. N Engl J Med 2012;366(16):1515–25.

4. Villasante Fricke AC, Miteva M. Epidemiology and burden of alopecia areata: a systematic review. Clin Cosmet Investig Dermatol 2015;8:397–403.

5. Rodriguez TA, Fernandes KE, Dresser KL, et al. Concordance rate of alopecia areata in identical twins supports both genetic and environmental factors. J Am Acad Dermatol 2010;62:525–7.

6. Alkhalifah A, et al. Alopecia areata update: part II. Treatment. J Am Acad Dermatol 2010;62(2):191–202 [quiz: 203–4].

7. Kang H, Wu W-Y, Lo BKK, et al. Hair follicles from alopecia areata patients exhibit alterations in immune privilege-associated gene expression in advance of hair loss. J Invest Dermatol 2010;130:2677–80.

8. Petukhova L, et al. Genome-wide association study in alopecia areata implicates both innate and adaptive immunity. Nature 2010;466(7302):113–7.

9. Cetin ED, et al. Investigation of the inflammatory mechanisms in alopecia areata. Am J Dermatopathol 2009;31(1):53–60.

10. Gregersen PK, Olsson LM. Recent advances in the genetics of autoimmune disease. Annu Rev Immunol 2009;27:363–91.

11. Paus R, et al. The hair follicle and immune privilege. J Investig Dermatol Symp Proc 2003;8(2):188–94.

12. Ito T, et al. Maintenance of hair follicle immune privilege is linked to prevention of NK cell attack. J Invest Dermatol 2008;128(5):1196–206.

13. Pender MP. CD8+ T-cell deficiency, Epstein-Barr virus infection, vitamin D deficiency, and steps to autoimmunity: a unifying hypothesis. Autoimmune Dis 2012;2012:189096.

14. Paus R, Bulfone-Paus S, Bertolini M. Hair follicle immune privilege revisited: the key to alopecia areata management. J Investig Dermatol Symp Proc 2018;19(1):S12–7.

15. Rawlings JS, Rosler DA, Harrison DA. The JAK/STAT signaling pathway. J Cell Sci 2004;117:1281–3.

16. Schwartz DM, et al. JAK inhibition as a therapeutic strategy for immune and inflammatory diseases. Nat Rev Drug Discov 2017;16(12):843–62.

17. Xing L, et al. Alopecia areata is driven by cytotoxic T lymphocytes and is reversed by JAK inhibition. Nat Med 2014;20(9):1043–9.

18. Mackay-Wiggan J, et al. Oral ruxolitinib induces hair regrowth in patients with moderate-to-severe alopecia areata. JCI Insight 2016;1(15):e89790.

19. Vandiver A, et al. Two cases of alopecia areata treated with ruxolitinib: a discussion of ideal dosing and laboratory monitoring. Int J Dermatol 2017;56(8):833–5.

20. Liu LY, King BA. Ruxolitinib for the treatment of severe alopecia areata. J Am Acad Dermatol 2019; 80(2):566–8.

21. Kennedy Crispin M, et al. Safety and efficacy of the JAK inhibitor tofacitinib citrate in patients with alopecia areata. JCI Insight 2016;1(15).

22. Liu LY, et al. Tofacitinib for the treatment of severe alopecia areata and variants: a study of 90 patients. J Am Acad Dermatol 2017;76(1):22–8.

23. Almutairi N, Nour TM, Hussain NH. Janus kinase inhibitors for the treatment of severe alopecia areata: an open-label comparative study. Dermatology 2019;235(2):130–6.

24. Castelo-Soccio L. Experience with oral tofacitinib in 8 adolescent patients with alopecia universalis. J Am Acad Dermatol 2017;76(4):754–5.

25. Craiglow BG, King BA. Tofacitinib for the treatment of alopecia areata in preadolescent children. J Am Acad Dermatol 2019;80(2):568–70.

26. Jabbari A, et al. Reversal of alopecia areata following treatment with the JAK1/2 inhibitor baricitinib. EBioMedicine 2015;2(4):351–5.

27. Olamiju B, Friedmann A, King B. Treatment of severe alopecia areata with baricitinib. J Am Acad Dermatol 2019;5(10):892–4.

28. Zhao H, Xu R, Huang XY, et al. Curcumin suppressed activation of dendritic cells via JAK/STAT/SOCS signal in mice with experimental colitis. Front Pharmacol 2016;7:455.

29. Putterman E, Castelo-Soccio L. Topical 2% tofacitinib for children with alopecia areata, alopecia totalis, and alopecia universalis. J Am Acad Dermatol 2018; 78(6):1207–9.

30. Bayart CB, et al. Topical Janus kinase inhibitors for the treatment of pediatric alopecia areata. J Am Acad Dermatol 2017;77(1):167–70.

31. Bokhari L, Sinclair RA-O. Treatment of alopecia universalis with topical Janus kinase inhibitors: a double blind, placebo, and active controlled pilot study. Int J Dermatol 2018;57(12):1464–70.

32. Deeb M, Beach RA. A case of topical ruxolitinib treatment failure in alopecia areata. J Cutan Med Surg 2017;21(6):562–3.

33. Mackay-Wiggan J, et al. An open-label study evaluating the efficacy of abatacept in alopecia areata. J Am Acad Dermatol 2021;84(3):841–4.

34. Trink A, et al. A randomized, double-blind, placebo- and active-controlled, half-head study to evaluate the effects of platelet-rich plasma on alopecia areata. Br J Dermatol 2013;169(3):690–4.

35. Li ZJ, et al. Autologous platelet-rich plasma: a potential therapeutic tool for promoting hair growth. Dermatol Surg 2012;38(7):1040–6.

36. Uebel CO, et al. The role of platelet plasma growth factors in male pattern baldness surgery. Plast Reconstr Surg 2006;118(6):1458–66.

37. El-Sharkawy H, et al. Platelet-rich plasma: growth factors and pro- and anti-inflammatory properties. J Peridontol 2007;78(4):661–9.

38. Shumez H, PP, Kaviarasan P, et al. Intralesional platelet rich plasma vs intralesional triamcinolone in the treatment of alopecia areata: a comparative study. Int J Med Res Health Sci 2015;4:118.

39. El Taieb MA, et al. Platelets rich plasma versus minoxidil 5% in treatment of alopecia areata: a trichoscopic evaluation. LID - 10.1111/dth.12437 [doi]. Dermatol Ther 2017;30(1). https://doi.org/10.1111/dth.12437.

40. Albalat W, Ebrahim HA-O. Evaluation of platelet-rich plasma vs intralesional steroid in treatment of alopecia areata. LID - 10.1111/jocd.12858 [doi]. J Cosmet Dermatol 2019;1473–2165. https://doi.org/10.1111/jocd.12858.

41. Mubki T. Platelet-rich plasma combined with intralesional triamcinolone acetonide for the treatment of alopecia areata: a case report. J Dermatol Surg 2016;20(1):87–90.

42. Darrigade AA-O, et al. Dual efficacy of dupilumab in a patient with concomitant atopic dermatitis and alopecia areata. Br J Dermatol 2018;179(2):534–6.

43. Uchida H, et al. Dupilumab improved alopecia areata in a patient with atopic dermatitis: a case report. Acta Dermatol Venereol 2019;99(7):675–6.

44. Penzi LR, et al. Hair regrowth in a patient with longstanding alopecia totalis and atopic dermatitis treated with dupilumab. JAMA Dermatol 2018; 154(11):1358–60.

Nutraceuticals

Glynis Ablon, MD

KEYWORDS

- Alopecia • Hair loss • Supplements • Nutrition • Nutraceuticals

KEY POINTS

- Several herbal products and vitamins have beneficial effects when used as oral supplements to treat hair loss.
- Numerous trials have demonstrated the clinical efficacy of proprietary nutraceutical products for treating hair loss in women and men.
- The overall safety of these nutraceuticals is very good.

INTRODUCTION

Although there are drugs approved by the US Food and Drug Administration for treating male and female pattern hair loss, some individuals are more comfortable using nonprescription medications. Frequently, they assume that these products are safer with fewer side effects than prescription drugs. Because the process of hair loss is affected by both intrinsic and extrinsic factors, companies are now expanding research efforts with the goal of creating natural supplements. In addition, they are combining over-the-counter ingredients to promote hair growth and regrowth for all forms of hair loss, including nonscarring and scarring alopecia.

It is increasingly clear that hair loss has a multifactorial etiology that includes an imbalance of the body's immune system and defects in several metabolic pathways. Internal triggers include diet and nutrition, the natural aging process, genetic hormones (dihydrotestosterone), and stress hormones (cortisol). External factors include extreme training and exercise, pollution, hair products and styling, and UV exposure. These triggers can cause an increase of free radicals, oxidative stress and microinflammation at the site of hair follicles. Combined, these factors can lead to dysregulation of complex follicle biology and immunology, as well as release of proapoptotic, profibrotic and proinflammatory cytokines and reactive oxygen species, all of which promote follicular regression, growth inhibition, and disruption of follicle stem cell cycling.[1-6] Because the hair follicle is closely regulated by very specific molecules released to initiate hair growth, regression, and rest, any disruption or dysregulation can tip the scale toward regression and hair loss.

The old adage, "you are what you eat" was never more appropriate than when discussing hair health. As individuals are living longer, it becomes increasingly important to understand the importance of diets rich in amino acids and certain botanicals, as well as the benefits of oral supplementation. The objective of this article was to describe the beneficial ingredients used to treat hair loss and the clinical evidence supporting their use.

HAIR SUPPLEMENT INGREDIENTS
Ashwagandha

This plant has its origins in Ayurvedic medicine used thousands of years ago, when it was thought to create balance in the body, increase energy, and improve stress resistance. Ashwagandha is an adaptogenic botanic containing steroidal lactones (withanolides) that can interact with steroid receptors by mimicking certain corticosteroids, thereby modulating cortisol levels and improving the stress response.[1,2]

Astaxanthin

Astaxanthin is a carotenoid that gives salmon and other seafood their pink color. As an antioxidant, it is 6000 times more potent than vitamin C, 550

UCLA Dermatology, 1600 Rosecrans Avenue, 4B, Manhattan Beach, CA 90266, USA
E-mail address: drablon@abloninstitute.com

Dermatol Clin 39 (2021) 417–427
https://doi.org/10.1016/j.det.2021.03.006

derm.theclinics.com

times more potent than green tea, and 550 times more potent than vitamin E.[3] Like all antioxidants, it decreases oxidative stress levels in mitochondria while decreasing proinflammatory cytokines such as IL-8.[4,5] Called the cell membrane antioxidant, it protects against oxidative mitochondrial dysfunction, allowing hair follicles to advance into growth cycle more readily. Oral astaxanthin is derived from the red algae *Haematococcus pluvialis* and it has been shown to improve the appearance of aging skin.[6,7]

Marine Collagen

Hydrolyzed marine collagen helps to build the structural integrity of the hair follicle and its environment. Hydrolyzing protein allows for lower molecular weight and better bioavailability, as well as improved diffusion of nutrients. It has been shown to have beneficial effects on aging skin.[8]

Turmeric (Curcuma longa)

Turmeric has anti-inflammatory, antimicrobial, antioxidant, and antineoplastic properties.[9] The active component of turmeric is curcumin, believed to be a 5α-reductase inhibitor that prevents conversion of testosterone to dihydrotestosterone. It inhibits nuclear factor-κB, proapoptotic inflammatory cytokines, tumor necrosis factor-alpha, and IL-1, which can induce follicular regression, as well as being(17–18 nutrafol reference) a free radical scavenger.[10] Oral and topical turmeric and curcumin products and supplements can provide therapeutic benefits for skin health.[11]

Red Clover (Trifolium pratense)

Red clover and other legumes are a rich source of the flavonoid biochanin A, a known inhibitor of 5α-reductase, which converts testosterone to 5α-dihydrotestosterone.[12]

Maca Root (Lepidium meyenii)

Maca root is found in Peru, where is has been cultured for centuries. It is a rich source of essential amino acids, fatty acids, and other nutrients, including vitamin C, copper, iron, and calcium.[13] Other constituents include glucosinolates, macamides, macaenes, alkaloids, and sterols.[14] The imidazole alkaloid lepidiline has been identified as the key active. It seems to improve the balance of endogenous sex hormones and increased fertility by its effect on 17β-hydroxysteroid dehydrogenase.[15] Maca root also has adaptogenic effects, reducing stress-induced elevated levels of corticosterone.[16] It may, therefore, help to decrease hair loss and miniaturization and increase hair growth.

Methylsulfonylmethane

Methylsulfonylmethane is widely found in food and beverages such as fruits, vegetables, grains, coffee, and cow's milk.[17] Methylsulfonylmethane has anti-inflammatory, antioxidant, and free radical scavenging activity and can modulate immune function.[17] A controlled study demonstrated methylsulfonylmethane significantly improved facial wrinkles, skin firmness, elasticity, and hydration.[18]

Amino Acids (L-cysteine, L-Methionine, and Taurine)

The most prevalent amino acids in keratin are L-cysteine and L-methionine, which are critical precursors for keratin hair protein synthesis. Because hair loss may be related to poor nutrition, it may be highly beneficial to provide supplemental amino acids.[19] Methionine has antioxidant activity that can protect protein[20] and is also vital for the synthesis of the precursor to collagen called procollagen. Additionally, cysteine is essential to produce the powerful antioxidant glutathione. Thus, cysteine also indirectly assists with protecting hair follicles from oxidative stress.

In vitro studies showed taurine is taken up by the connective tissue sheath, proximal outer root sheath, and hair bulb and promoted hair survival preventing transforming growth factor-beta1–induced damage on hair follicles.[21] Several studies have confirmed that cysteine supplementation can decrease the symptoms of androgenic alopecia.[22]

Piperine (Piper nigrum)

Piperine is derived from black pepper. It has significant and dose-dependent immunomodulating, anti-inflammatory, antioxidant, and anticancer activity.[23,24] Piperine has demonstrated 5α-reductase inhibitory activity and increased hair growth in an animal model.[25] It possesses direct antioxidant activity against various free radicals, protecting tissues from peroxidative damage.[26] Piperine can also enhance the bioavailability of other nutraceuticals. For example, it can increase the antioxidant, anti-inflammatory, antimicrobial, and antineoplastic effects of curcumin.[27]

Saw Palmetto (Serenoa repens)

Saw palmetto is derived from the fruit of a small palm tree. It inhibits 5α-reductase and prevents the conversion of testosterone to dihydrotestosterone.[28] A small placebo-controlled, double-blind study assessed the benefit of saw palmetto for treating androgenetic alopecia.[29] The results demonstrated that 60% of study patients dosed with the active study formulation were rated as improved.

Horsetail (Equisetum spp.)

An extract from 1 species of horsetail has been shown to have high inhibitory activity against 5α-reductase, IL-6 secretion, and lipid peroxidation.[30]

Minerals (Iron and Zinc)

Iron deficiency is the most common nutritional deficiency[31] and is common among women with hair loss.[32,33] Iron supplementation is indicated in patients with iron or ferritin deficiency and hair loss.[31] Zinc deficiency is also associated with hair loss, which can be reversed with zinc supplementation.[34] In 1 study, 66.7% of patients with alopecia areata and low zinc levels responded to treatment with zinc gluconate supplementation.[35]

Vitamins

Because vitamins play an essential role in the hair cycle and immune defense system, hair loss can occur as a result of nutrient deficiency.[36,37] These include vitamins A, B, C (ascorbic acid, acerola), D, E (tocotrienols), biotin, and folic acid. Patients with alopecia have shown lower levels of endogenous antioxidants and an increase in metabolites of lipid peroxidation.[38] Tocotrienols decrease oxidative stress and prevent lipid peroxidation secondary to their superior lipid solubility. Although a link can be demonstrated between some vitamin deficiency and hair loss, the ability of vitamin supplementation to restore hair is less clear.[31]

PROPRIETARY SUPPLEMENTS FOR HAIR LOSS

Several companies have combined these nutritional ingredients to create unique and effective supplements for treating hair loss. In a largely unregulated supplement industry, it is as difficult for physicians as it is for patients to discern clinical efficacy, standardization of dosing, or clean sourcing of ingredients. These nutraceuticals contain ingredients that work on multiple levels of intrinsic and extrinsic causes of hair loss. The following clinical data support the use of these products.

Nutrafol

Ingredients

- Ashwaganda
- Biocurcumin
- Tocotrienols
- Saw palmetto
- Piperine
- Marine collagen

Nutrafol is a nutraceutical supplement with 3 core formulations, all of which contain a proprietary complex of highly purified, bio-optimized botanicals containing exact standardized dosages of phytoactives with shown multimodal clinical efficacy against dihydrotestosterone, inflammation, reactive oxygen species, mediators of psychoemotional stress, and intermediary signaling cascades.[39,40] Nutrafol took advantage of advances in biotechnology, using solvent-free methods to extract the most potent photoactive plant parts and standardizing them to specific dosages, while bio-optimizing for improved bioavailability and absorption.

Nutrafol's formulations are personalized based on age and sex. The 3 core formulations include Men's, Women's and Women's Balance, which is the most recent formulation for women in perimenopause, menopause, and after menopause. The men's and women's formulas contain a signature Synergen Complex with ingredients specifically selected based on their pharmacology and multimodal activity against the multiple molecular and environmental causative factors of hair loss, described in detail by Farris and colleagues in 2017.[39]

Patients with alopecia have been shown to have lower levels of endogenous antioxidants and an increase in metabolites of lipid peroxidation.[38] Several botanic ingredients in Nutrafol formulations have antioxidant properties. The tocotrienol-rich tocotrienol/tocopherol complex in the Synergen Complex was clinically shown to improve hair growth, likely by reducing oxidative stress in the scalp.[39,41,42] A unique feature in all Nutrafol formulations is the addition of phytoactive stress adaptogens, presenting the only available option for addressing psychoemotional stress and its impact on hair follicles.[39,43] Sensoril ashwagandha in Nutrafol formulations is standardized to a higher percentage of withanolides and was shown clinically to significantly decrease elevated cortisol levels in chronically stressed adults with daily administration.[44]

The Women's Balance formula contains Synergen Complex plus, which is optimized with dosages and additional ingredients that specifically address the hormonal and oxidative changes that occur during the menopausal transition in life and afterward. The hair follicle is sensitive not only to androgens, but also to estrogens, progesterone, and the ratios of these numerous hormones relative to each other. Decrease in estrogen during menopause is associated with a decreased rate of hair growth, hair diameter and density, as well as percentage of anagen hairs.[45] Although estrogen and progesterone decrease rapidly after menopause, levels of androgens decrease slowly, resulting in a relative androgen dominance—an imbalance that contributes to the increased appearance of hair loss during this time in women.[46] To counter the extra effects of androgens during menopause in women, Women's Balance is formulated with significantly more saw palmetto. Additional ingredients include organic maca root and astaxanthin. Traditionally known for its hormone balancing properties, maca is likewise an adaptogen that helps modulate the hypothalamic–pituitary–ovary axis through a variety of clinically shown effects on production of endogenous sex hormones.[40,43,47] In a clinical trial, the administration of maca to perimenopausal women for 2 months significantly improved endogenous production of estrogen, follicle-stimulating hormone, progesterone, and adrenocorticotrophic hormone levels, as well as mitigated menopausal symptoms.[47] Astaxanthin is a very potent antioxidant derived from micro algae and included in the formulation to support against age-related decrease in antioxidant defense mechanisms and increased oxidative stress in postmenopausal women.[48]

The efficacy of Nutrafol's complete formulations has been clinically tested in published and ongoing studies. In a recent randomized, double-blind, placebo-controlled trial, daily intake of Nutrafol Women's capsules was shown to significantly improve several hair growth and hair quality parameters in women with self-perceived thinning.

In this 6-month randomized, double-blind, placebo-controlled study, enrolled patients were randomized to receive Nutrafol or placebo for 90 days. The primary end point in this study was the change in the number of terminal and vellus hairs based on phototrichograms obtained through macrophotography analysis of an area of the scalp. Daily administration of Nutrafol increased the baseline number of terminal and vellus hairs in the target area at days 90 and 180 to a significantly greater extent than placebo. A blinded investigator assessment revealed significant improvements in hair growth and overall hair quality. A significant percentage of patients taking Nutrafol also reported improvement in hair growth, volume, thickness, and hair growth rate, as well as decreased anxiety and other wellness parameters. There were no reports of adverse events.

A recently published collection of case reports demonstrated that the efficacy of Nutrafol Women's formula alone or in combination with other regimens is showing success without ethnic barriers, specifically in darker skin types of African descent.[49] In a mixed ethnicity study of 87 men and women of Caucasian, Asian, African American, and Hispanic descent, taking respective Nutrafol Men and Nutrafol Women capsules, a significant percent saw improvement in scalp coverage and thickness of hair, as well as other parameters like less shedding and growth. Specifically, 75% of the African American group saw improved hair growth and thickness after 6 months of daily use.[50] In a study of 30 women with self-perceived hair thinning in perimenopause, during menopause, and after menopause, daily administration of Nutrafol Women's Balance resulted in 73% seeing more scalp coverage and less shedding by 6 months, which increased to 80% and 90% by 9 months, respectively. Furthermore, 80% saw new hair growth by 6 months, increasing to 93% by 9 months. Additionally, 90% reported improvement in texture by 9 months. The phytoactives in Nutrafol have preserved bioactivity after traction with solvents that are bioavailable to the body and free of additives and toxins.

An interim analysis of a 6-month randomized placebo-controlled study was completed recently. The results showed that the daily intake of the nutraceutical supplement resulted in statistically significant improvements for the active treatment group for the number of terminal, vellus, and total hairs and hair shedding after 90 days and further improvement after 180 days (for each, $P<.005$) among women going through menopausal transition.[51] A representative male patient is shown at baseline and after 6 months of treatment in **Fig. 1**. A female patient is shown after treatment at 3 and 6 months in **Fig. 2**.

Viviscal

Ingredients

- AminoMar (28% marine protein complex)
- L-Cysteine and L-methionine
- Vitamin C
- Apple extract (procyanidin B_2)
- Biotin
- Fumed silica

After studying the Innuits, a Scandinavian professor determined their excellent skin and hair quality was the result of their fish- and protein-rich diet, leading to the development of a marine protein-derived proprietary hair thickening supplement. The beneficial effects of this product have been documented in numerous in vitro studies and clinical trials.

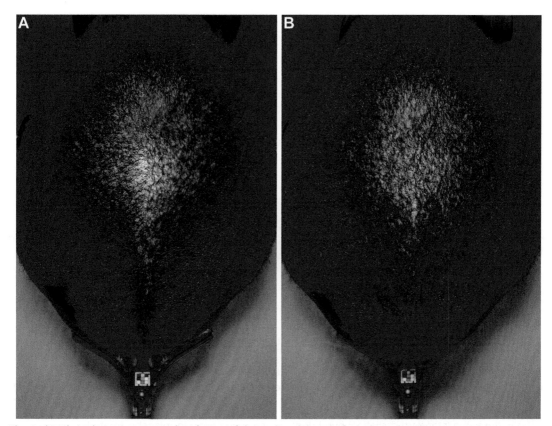

Fig. 1. (*A*, *B*). Male patient treated with Nutrafol. Baseline (*A*) and after 6 months of treatment (*B*).

Viviscal is an oral marine supplement designed to promote hair growth in women with temporary thinning hair (Viviscal Ltd, Ewing, NJ). This product comprises the key ingredients AminoMar C marine complex (a proprietary blend of shark and mollusk powder derived from sustainable marine sources), *Equisetum arvense* (a naturally occurring form of silica), *Malpighia glabra* (acerola cherry providing vitamin C), biotin, and zinc.

Studies of the dermal papilla, or control center of the hair follicle, demonstrate cell proliferation and cell signaling triggered by Viviscal, leading to a new anagen growth phase. Doubling the alkaline phosphatase in each dermal papilla helps to support healthy hair growth and increased cellular communication.

Viviscal originated as products containing glycosaminoglycans extracted from marine fish[52] and cartilage polysaccharides.[53] Two early double-blind studies assessed the beneficial effects of these ingredients in women with photodamaged skin.[52,53] In addition to improvements in skin quality, there were improvements in hair and nails. A subsequent double-blind study specifically assessed the effects marine extracts and a silica compound on men with androgenic

alopecia.[54] Patients treated with the oral supplement achieved a mean 38% increase in nonvellus hairs and 95% showed a clinical and histologic cure.

The initial study with the current Viviscal formulation was an open-label pilot study.[55] Female patients with self-perceived thinning hair associated with poor diet, stress, hormonal influences, or abnormal menstrual cycles were enrolled. At baseline, the mean number of shed hairs was 69.1, decreasing to 61.0 and 37.0 after 4 and 10 weeks of treatment, respectively.[55] At week 10, most patients reported beneficial effects in overall hair volume, scalp coverage, hair thickness, softness, shine, decreased hair shedding, and improved overall skin health.

Based on these positive results, several randomized, placebo-controlled, double-blind studies further evaluated the ability of Viviscal to increase hair growth using objective measures. In the first study, healthy adult women with self-perceived thinning hair were randomized to receive Viviscal or placebo twice daily for 180 days.[56] A 2 cm^2 area of scalp was selected for hair counts at baseline and after 90 and 180 days of treatment. Among Viviscal-treated

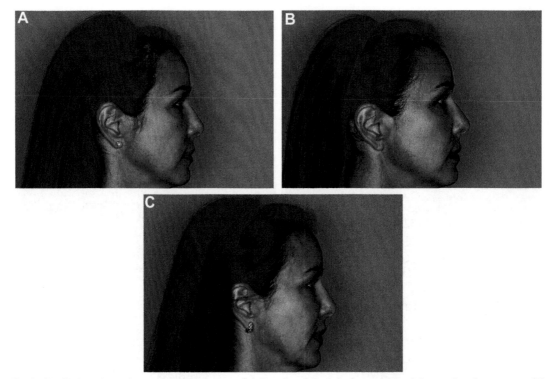

Fig. 2. (*A–C*). Female patient treated with Nutrafol. Baseline (*A*) and after 3 (*B*) and 6 months of treatment (*C*).

patients, the mean (standard deviation) number of baseline terminal hairs was 271.0 (24.2) at baseline, increasing to 571 (65.7) and 609.6 (66.6) after 90 and 180 days of treatment, respectively, while remaining essentially unchanged among patients treated with placebo.[56] Viviscal-treated patients reported significantly greater improvements in overall hair volume, scalp coverage, and hair body thickness after 90 days and also hair shine and skin smoothness after 180 days.

The results of 2 other double-blind, placebo-controlled studies confirmed the ability of Viviscal to promote hair growth and increase hair diameter in larger cohorts of women with self-perceived thinning hair.[57,58] In each study, healthy adult women were enrolled and randomized to receive Viviscal or placebo every morning and evening and were evaluated at baseline and after 90 days[57] or 90 and 180 days of treatment.[7] An area of scalp was again selected for phototricho-gram analysis. Among patients treated with the active product, there was a significant increase in the mean standard deviation number of terminal hairs from 178.3 (7.8) at baseline to 235.8 (18.4) after 90 days[57] and from 189.9 (15.2) at baseline to 297.4 (96.1) and 341.0 (60.9) at 90 and 180 days, respectively.[58] Similarly, there was a significant increase in the number of vellus hairs in patients receiving Viviscal.[57,58] In contrast, there were no

improvements in placebo-treated patients. Improvements in a 90-day self-assessment questionnaire included overall hair growth and hair volume, scalp coverage, thickness of hair body, hair strength, growth of eyebrow hair, and overall skin health.[57,58] Viviscal also produced improvements in a 180-day self-assessment questionnaire and quality of life questionnaire.[58]

An additional 180-day double-blind, placebo-controlled study added a shed hair count analysis and a phototrichogram-based hair fiber diameter analysis as efficacy end points.[59] An area of the scalp was again selected for 2-dimensional digital images and trichoanalysis. Patients were randomized to receive 1 tablet of the active treatment or a placebo 3 times daily and evaluated at baseline and after 2 days and 3 and 6 months of treatment. Among patients randomized to Viviscal, mean hair shedding was significantly reduced from 52.1 (59.5) at baseline to 42.6 (45.2) at 3 months and 42.7 (41.7) at 6 months. The mean hair diameter of vellus-like hair showed a small but significant increase among patients treated with Viviscal after 3 and 6 months of treatment. There was no improvement among placebo-treated patients. Improvements after 6 months of treatment are apparent in the patient shown in **Fig. 3**.

The beneficial effects of Viviscal for restoring thinning hair has also been demonstrated in other

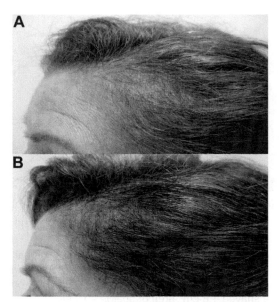

Fig. 3. (*A, B*) Female patient treated with Viviscal. Baseline (*A*) and after and 6 months of treatment (*B*).

patient populations, including men. A double-blind, placebo-controlled study assessed the beneficial effects of a new formulation for men.[60] Healthy patients with thinning hair, including individuals with androgenic alopecia were randomized to receive Viviscal Man or placebo every morning and evening and were evaluated at baseline and post-treatment days 90 and 180. **Fig. 4** demonstrates improvements in a male patient after 3 and 6 months of treatment.

Like previous studies, a predesignated target area on the scalp was chosen for digital imaging and trichoanalysis. This study introduced the hair pull test,[61] which was performed on the right and left parietal, frontal, and occipital areas of the scalp at baseline and the day 180 visits. The mean (standard deviation) total hair count significantly increased from 162.2 (46.9) at baseline to 169.1 (43.4) and 174.9 (44.0) at days 90 and 180, respectively; the total hair density significantly increased from 159.7 (46.3) at baseline to 166.5 (42.7) and 172.2 (43.3) at days 90 and 180, respectively; the terminal hair density significantly increased from 121.9 (40.0) at baseline to 127.7 (39.21) and 130.3 (38.8) at days 90 and 180, respectively; and the hair pull test was significantly improved at days 90 and 180. There was no improvement in placebo-treated patients. Post-treatment questionnaires revealed significant overall improvement in quality of life and substantial overall satisfaction at day 180.

In an open-label study, the effects of Viviscal were also assessed in women of color.[62] Study

patients with scarring alopecia, traction alopecia, or self-perceived thinning hair were treated with Viviscal twice daily and were evaluated at baseline and after 2 and 4 months of treatment.

Baseline quality of life questionnaires indicated the effects of thinning hair include embarrassment and diminished self-esteem. Substantial improvements were observed during the initial 2 months of treatment. Based on patient self-assessments, these changes included overall hair volume, scalp coverage, thickness of hair body, hair shine, and daily number of lost hairs.

Throughout these clinical studies, Viviscal demonstrated an excellent safety profile.

Lambdapil

Ingredients

- Saw palmetto
- L-cystine
- Biotin
- Taurine
- Zinc
- Sillicium (horsetail dry extract)
- Vitamins B_3, B_5, and B_6

A single randomized, double-blind, placebo-controlled trial assessed the efficacy of Lambdapil capsules for treating hair loss in female and male patients.[63] Enrolled patients had confirmed telogen effluvium or androgenetic alopecia and were randomized to receive Lambdapil or placebo twice daily for 6 months. Product efficacy was assessed using the hair pull test, phototrichogram procedure on a chosen area of scalp, and digital macrophotography. Hair volume and appearance were assessed by a dermatologist using a 7-point clinical score scale and patients responded to self-assessment questionnaires.

To perform the hair pull test, gentle traction is applied to a cluster of approximately 60 hairs on different areas and the number of extracted hairs is counted. In this study, the test was performed frontal, temporal, and occipital areas of the scalp. Growing anagen hairs should remain rooted, whereas telogen hairs come out easily. Normally, fewer than 3 telogen-phase hairs should come out with each pull; however, a loss of more than 9 hairs suggests telogen effluvium.

The number of hairs removed in the pull test decreased steadily for both groups, but was significantly less for the Lambdapil-treated group after 1 month. Among men, there was a significant 23.4% increase in the baseline anagen/telogen ratio in the Lambdapil group and which was significantly greater than placebo-treated patients. Among both women and men, most reported a

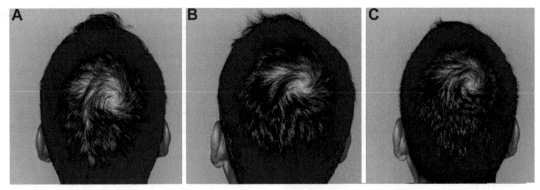

Fig. 4. (*A–C*) Male patient treated with Viviscal. Baseline (*A*) and after 3 months (*B*) and 6 months of treatment (*C*).

slight or moderate increase in hair volume, which was significantly greater in the Lambdapil group beginning at month 3 and month 6 (**Fig. 5**). Results from a quality of life questionnaire showed an improvement in baseline scores the Lambdapil-treated group, which was significant at 3 months. In contrast, quality of life scores decreased in the placebo group. Overall, Lambdapil-treated patients noticed a greater improvement in indicators of hair growth compared with the placebo group.

HRS-10 Hair Regrowth System

Ingredients

- Biomimetic peptide (acetyl tetrapeptide-3)
- Red clover extract (biochanin A)

To assess the clinical efficacy of this product, 30 healthy volunteers with mild-to-moderate hair loss enrolled in a 4-month randomized, placebo-controlled study.[64] As an inclusion criterion, less than 70% of all hair were required to be in the anagen phase. Patients were randomized to receive the medicated hair lotion containing clover extract (15 ppm biochanin A) and 300 ppm acetyl tetrapeptide-3 or placebo. Patients applied 20 drops of their assigned treatment to balding areas and gently massage it into the entire scalp. Each week, patients were provided a plastic bag to collect all hair found on their pillow, comb, and clothes each day, which was returned for hair counts. Efficacy was objectively assessed using a digital trichogram and total hair density was on a shaved 1.8 cm^2 area of scalp.

Treatment with the test product significantly increased anagen hair density after 4 months of treatment, whereas there was no change among placebo-treated patients. The number of hairs in the anagen phase increased by a mean of 13% in the treated group versus a 2% decrease in the placebo group. The test product also decreased the mean telogen hair density by 29% versus a 23% increase in the placebo group. Accordingly, the baseline anagen/telogen ration significantly increased by 46% in the treated group while significantly decreasing by 33% in the placebo group. The overall tolerability of the topical formulations was excellent; no adverse events were reported.

Noncommercial Supplement

Ingredients

- Fish oil 460 mg
- Blackcurrant seed oil 460 mg
- Vitamin E 5 mg
- Vitamin C 30 mg
- Lycopene 1 mg

This 6-month, randomized, single-blind study assessed the efficacy of a nutritional supplement

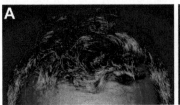
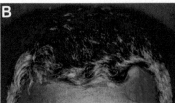
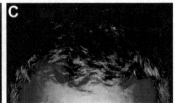

Fig. 5. (*A–C*). Male patient treated with Lambdapil. Baseline (*A*) and after 3 months (*B*) and 6 months of treatment (*C*).

on patients with Ludwig stage 1 hair loss.[65] Control patients did not receive any product. The primary efficacy measure was change in hair density based on global digital images. The trichogram method was used to study hair loss and distribution of hair diameter. A self-assessment questionnaire queried patients about hair loss, hair density, and hair shaft condition (hair diameter, shiny appearance, volume, and softness) after 3 and 6 months.

After 6 months, 62.0% of treated patients had increased hair versus 28.2% in the control group. Improvement in hair density among treated patients was also significantly better in than control patients. At the end of the study, 88.6% of patients in the supplement group reported increased hair density of their scalp described as slight (13.9%), moderate (45.6%), and large (29.1%) versus 51.3% among control patients. The percentage of telogen hair decreased in both groups, but significantly more in treated patients. The proportion of nonvellus anagen hair was 79.7% at baseline increasing to 87.7% after 6 months versus no change in control patients. A significant increase in trichometer index at 6 months indicated an increase in hair density and thickness. All patients reported improvements in all assessment parameters and overall satisfaction was 92.4%.

SUMMARY

There are a variety of products used for hair growth. Some require a prescription, but many do not. As the science of hair growth advances and the demand for new products increases, it is likely that we will see many more products that will be marketed for hair regrowth.

DISCLOSURE

Nutrafol: Clinical Research Investigator; Viviscal: Clinical Research Investigator.

REFERENCES

1. Bhattacharya SK, Gorl GR, Kaur R, et al. Anti-stress activity of Sitoindosides VII and VIII. New acylsteryl-glucosides from Withania somnifera. Phytother Res 1987;1:32–7.
2. Chandrasekhar K, Kapoor J, Anishetty S. A prospective, randomized double-blind, placebo-controlled study of safety and efficacy of a high-concentration full-spectrum extract of ashwagandha root in reducing stress and anxiety in adults. Indian J Psychol Med 2012;34:255–62.
3. Ekpe L, Inaku K, Ekpe V. Antioxidant effects of astaxanthin in various diseases—a review. J Mol Pathophysiol 2018;7:1–6.
4. Kim SH, Lim JW, Kim H. Astaxanthin inhibits mitochondrial dysfunction and interleukin-8 expression in Helicobacter pylori-infected gastric epithelial cells. Nutrients 2018;10:E1320.
5. Pashkow FJ, Watumull DG, Campbell CL. Astaxanthin: a novel potential treatment for oxidative stress and inflammation in cardiovascular disease. Am J Cardiol 2008;101:58–68D.
6. Tominaga K, Hongo N, Karato M, et al. Cosmetic benefits of astaxanthin on human subjects. Acta Biochim Pol 2012;59:43–7.
7. Ng QX, De Deyn MLZQ, Loke W, et al. Effects of astaxanthin supplementation on skin health: a systematic review of clinical studies. J Diet Suppl 2020;23: 1–14.
8. Proksch E, Segger D, Degwert J, et al. Oral supplementation of specific collagen peptides has beneficial effects on human skin physiology: a double-blind, placebo-controlled study. Skin Pharmacol Physiol 2014;27:47–55.
9. Hewlings SJ, Kalman DS. Curcumin: a review of its effects on human health. Foods 2017;6:92.
10. Tomren MA, Másson M, Loftsson T, et al. Studies on curcumin and curcuminoids XXXI. Symmetric and asymmetric curcuminoids: stability, activity and complexation with cyclodextrin. Int J Pharm 2007; 338:27–34.
11. Vaughn AR, Branum A, Sivamani RK. Effects of turmeric (Curcuma longa) on skin health: a systematic review of the clinical evidence. Phytother Res 2016;30:1243–64.
12. Hiipakka RA, Zhang HZ, Dai W, et al. Structure-activity relationships for inhibition of human 5alpha-reductases by polyphenols. Biochem Pharmacol 2002;63:1165–76.
13. da Silva Leitão Peres N, Cabrera Parra Bortoluzzi L, Medeiros Marques LL, et al. Medicinal effects of Peruvian maca (Lepidium meyenii): a review. Food Funct 2020;11:83–92.
14. Huang YJ, Peng XR, Qiu MH. Progress on the chemical constituents derived from glucosinolates in maca (Lepidium meyenii). Nat Prod Bioprospect 2018;8:405–12.
15. Cheng C, Shen F, Ding G, et al. Lepidiline A improves the balance of endogenous sex hormones and increases fecundity by targeting HSD17B1. Mol Nutr Food Res 2020;64(10):e1900706.
16. López-Fando A, Gómez-Serranillos MP, Iglesias I, et al. Lepidium peruvianum chacon restores homeostasis impaired by restraint stress. Phytother Res 2004;18:471–4.
17. Butawan M, Benjamin RL, Bloomer RJ. Methylsulfonylmethane: applications and safety of a novel dietary supplement. Nutrients 2017;9:E290.
18. Muizzuddin N, Benjamin R. Beauty from within: oral administration of a sulfur-containing supplement methylsulfonylmethane improves signs of skin

ageing. Int J Vitam Nutr Res 2020;1–10. https://doi. org/10.1024/0300-9831/a000643.

19. Goluch-Koniuszy ZS. Nutrition of women with hair loss problem during the period of menopause. Prz Menopauzalny 2016;15:56–61.

20. Luo S, Levine RL. Methionine in proteins defends against oxidative stress. FASEB J 2009;23:464–72.

21. Collin C, Gautier B, Gaillard O, et al. Protective effects of taurine on human hair follicle grown in vitro. Int J Cosmet Sci 2006;28:289–98.

22. Blumeyer A, Tosti A, Messenger A, et al. Evidence-based (S3) guideline for the treatment of androgenetic alopecia in women and in men. J Dtsch Dermatol Ges 2011;9:S1–57.

23. Smilkov K, Ackova DG, Cvetkovski A, et al. Piperine: old spice and new nutraceutical? Curr Pharm Des 2019;25:1729–39.

24. Meghwal M, Goswami TK. Piper nigrum and piperine: an update. Phytother Res 2013;27: 1121–30.

25. Hirata N, Tokunaga M, Naruto S, et al. Testosterone 5alpha-reductase inhibitory active constituents of Piper nigrum leaf. Biol Pharm Bull 2007;30:2402–5.

26. Mittal R, Gupta RL. In vitro antioxidant activity of piperine. Methods Find Exp Clin Pharmacol 2000; 22:271–4.

27. Shoba G, Joy D, Joseph T, et al. Influence of piperine on the pharmacokinetics of curcumin in animals and human volunteers. Planta Med 1998;64: 353–6.

28. Buonocore D, Verri M, Cattaneo L, et al. Serenoa repens extracts: in vitro study of the 5α-reductase activity in a co-culture model for benign prostatic hyperplasia. Arch Ital Urol Androl 2018;90:199–202.

29. Prager N, Bickett K, French N, et al. A randomized, double-blind, placebo-controlled trial to determine the effectiveness of botanically derived inhibitors of 5-alpha-reductase in the treatment of androgenetic alopecia. J Altern Complement Med 2002;8: 143–52.

30. Chaiyana W, Punyoyai C, Somwongin S, et al. Inhibition of 5α-reductase, IL-6 secretion, and oxidation process of Equisetum debile Roxb. ex vaucher extract as functional food and nutraceuticals ingredients. Nutrients 2017;9:E1105.

31. Almohanna HM, Ahmed AA, Tsatalis JP, et al. The role of vitamins and minerals in hair loss: a review. Dermatol Ther (Heidelb) 2019;9:51–70.

32. St Pierre SA, Vercellotti GM, Donovan JC, et al. Iron deficiency and diffuse nonscarring scalp alopecia in women: more pieces to the puzzle. J Am Acad Dermatol 2010;63:1070–6.

33. Rushton DH. Nutritional factors and hair loss. Clin Exp Dermatol 2002;27:396–404.

34. Alhaj E, Alhaj N, Alhaj NE. Diffuse alopecia in a child due to dietary zinc deficiency. Skinmed 2007;6: 199–200.

35. Park H, Kim CW, Kim SS, et al. The therapeutic effect and the changed serum zinc level after zinc supplementation in alopecia areata patients who had a low serum zinc level. Ann Dermatol 2009;21:142–6.

36. Strumia R. Dermatologic signs in patients with eating disorders. Am J Clin Dermatol 2005;6: 165–73.

37. Cheung EJ, Sink JR, English JC. Vitamin and mineral deficiencies in patients with telogen effluvium: a retrospective cross-sectional study. J Drugs Dermatol 2016;15:1235–7.

38. Naziroglu M, Kokcam I. Antioxidants and lipid peroxidation status in the blood of patients with alopecia. Cell Biochem Funct 2000;18:169–73.

39. Farris PK, Rogers N, McMichael A, et al. A novel multi-targeting approach to treating hair loss, using standardized nutraceuticals. J Drugs Dermatol 2017;16:s141–8.

40. Ablon G, Kogan S. A six-month, randomized, double-blind, placebo-controlled study evaluating the safety and efficacy of a nutraceutical supplement for promoting hair growth in women with self-perceived thinning hair. J Drugs Dermatol 2018;17:558–65.

41. Beoy LA, Woei WJ, Hay YK. Effects of tocotrienol supplementation on hair growth in human volunteers. Trop Life Sci Res 2010;21:91–9.

42. Wang Y, Park NY, Jang Y, et al. Vitamin E gamma-tocotrienol inhibits cytokine-stimulated NF-kappaB activation by induction of anti-Inflammatory A20 via stress adaptive response due to modulation of sphingolipids. J Immunol 2015;195:126–33.

43. Sadick NS, Callender VD, Kircik LH, et al. New insight into the pathophysiology of hair loss trigger a paradigm shift in the treatment approach. J Drugs Dermatol 2017;16:s135–40.

44. Auddy B, Hazra J, Mitra A, et al. A standardized Withania somnifera extract significantly reduces stress-related parameters in chronically stressed humans: a double-blind, randomized, placebo-controlled study. JANA 2008;11:50–66.

45. Mirmirani P. Hormonal changes in menopause: do they contribute to a 'midlife hair crisis' in women? Br J Dermatol 2011;165:7–11.

46. Markopoulos MC, Kassi E, Alexandraki KI, et al. Hyperandrogenism after menopause. Eur J Endocrinol 2015;172:R79–91.

47. Meissner HO, Kapczynski W, Mscisz A, et al. Use of gelatinized maca (lepidium peruvianum) in early postmenopausal women. Int J Biomed Sci 2005;1: 33–45.

48. Miquel J, Ramírez-Boscá A, Ramírez-Bosca JV, et al. Menopause: a review on the role of oxygen stress and favorable effects of dietary antioxidants. Arch Gerontol Geriatr 2006;42:289–306.

49. Burgess C, Roberts W, Downie J, et al. A closer look at a multi-targeted approach to hair loss in African American women. J Drugs Dermatol 2020;19:95–8.

50. Data on file. Nutraceutical Wellness, Inc; 2020.

51. Data on file. New York: Nutraceutical Wellness Inc.

52. Lassus A, Eskanen L, Happonen HP, et al. Imedeen for the treatment of degenerated skin in females. J Int Med Res 1991;19:147–52.

53. Eskelinin A, Santalahti J. Special natural cartilage polysaccharides for the treatment of sun-damaged skin in females. J Int Med Res 1992;20:99–105.

54. Lassus A, Eskelinen E. A comparative study of a new food supplement, ViviScal, with fish extract for the treatment of hereditary androgenic alopecia in young males. J Int Med Res 1992;20:445–53.

55. Murphy J. A 10-week pilot consumer perception test to evaluate the overall acceptability of a Viviscal oral supplement when used by females with self-perceived thinning hair. 2010. Available at: http://www.viviscal.com/media//cms/docs/pilot-study.pdf. Accessed August, 2016.

56. Ablon G. A double-blind, placebo-controlled study evaluating the efficacy of an oral supplement in women with self-perceived thinning hair. J Clin Aesthet Dermatol 2012;5:28–34.

57. Ablon G. A 3-month, randomized, double-blind, placebo-controlled study evaluating the ability of an extra-strength marine protein supplement to promote hair growth and decrease shedding in women with self-perceived thinning hair. Dermatol Res Pract 2015;2015:841570.

58. Ablon G, Dayan S. A randomized, double-blind, placebo-controlled, multi-center, extension trial evaluating the efficacy of a new oral supplement in women with self-perceived thinning hair. J Clin Aesthet Dermatol 2015;8:15–21.

59. Rizer RL, Stephens TJ, Herndon JH, et al. A marine protein-based dietary supplement for subclinical hair thinning/loss: results of a multisite, double-blind, placebo-controlled clinical trial. Int J Trichology 2015;7:156–66.

60. Ablon G. A 6-month, randomized, double-blind, placebo-controlled study evaluating the ability of a marine complex supplement to promote hair growth in men with thinning hair. J Cosmet Dermatol 2016; 15:358–66.

61. Shapiro J, Wiseman M, Lui H. Practical management of hair loss. Can Fam Physician 2000;46:1469–77.

62. Jackson B. A 4-month clinical study evaluating the efficacy and tolerability of an oral supplement for the treatment of thinning hair in African American women. South Beach Symposium; February 2011; Miami Beach, FL.

63. Narda M, Aladren S, Cestone E, et al. Extract and biotin for hair loss in healthy males and females. A prospective, randomized, double-blinded, controlled clinical trial. J Cosmo Trichol 2017;3:1–8.

64. Loing E, Lachance R, Ollier V, et al. A new strategy to modulate alopecia using a combination of two specific and unique ingredients. J Cosmet Sci 2013;64:45–58.

65. Le Floc'h C, Cheniti A, Connétable S, et al. Effect of a nutritional supplement on hair loss in women. J Cosmet Dermatol 2015;14:76–82.

Platelet-rich Plasma and Cell Therapy
The New Horizon in Hair Loss Treatment

Aditya K. Gupta, MD, PhD[a,b,]*, Helen J. Renaud, PhD[b],
Jeffrey A. Rapaport, MD[c]

KEYWORDS

• Platelet-rich plasma • Cell therapy • Exosomes • Androgenetic alopecia • Alopecia areata

KEY POINTS

• Platelet-rich plasma (PRP) is efficacious in treating androgenetic alopecia (AGA) and alopecia areata (AA), especially in mild to moderate clinical cases in men.
• Evidence to support cell-based therapies for treatment of AGA and AA is promising but limited as research in this field is in its infancy.
• Preparation of PRP and cell-based therapies varies widely between studies. Standardization of preparation techniques is needed.
• Standardization of treatment dose and regimen is needed for both PRP and cell-based therapies.
• Larger, prospective, randomized studies are needed to validate the reported efficacies of PRP and cell-based therapies.

INTRODUCTION

Treating patients with hair loss presents a unique challenge to the physician. Hair loss is a common affliction in both men and women and can have a negative impact on self-confidence and self-worth.[1] Despite the prevalence and negative psychological impact on the patient, however, a valid cure does not exist and the current medicinal therapies have limited effectiveness making hair loss a persisting, unsolved problem.

The most common type of nonscarring hair loss is androgenetic alopecia (AGA), also known as male pattern or female pattern hair loss,[2] and manifests as progressive hair follicle miniaturization.[3] The current US Food and Drug Administration (FDA)-approved medical treatments for AGA, finasteride and minoxidil, are effective at arresting hair loss progression, but they fall short of promoting hair regrowth. Additionally, they require persistent, indefinite use to maintain hair density and can

have unwanted adverse effects, leaving patients frustrated and dissatisfied. Low-level laser therapy, an FDA-cleared treatment for AGA, has shown promising results; however, the effectiveness of this treatment still is debated.[4,5] Surgical hair transplantation is a more permanent option but is an invasive procedure and comes with a high monetary cost, which deters many patients. This dearth in treatment options has prompted the search for alternative treatments for AGA that are effective, safe, and scientifically sound.

Another encountered form of nonscarring hair loss is alopecia areata (AA), which is an autoimmune disorder. Significant variation in the clinical presentation of AA ranges from well-circumscribed patches of hair loss to complete absence of body and scalp hair. AA affects all age groups and ethnicities as well as both genders. The lifetime risk is estimated at 2%.[6] The cause of AA is not understood completely, but loss of immune privilege in the hair follicle leading to autoimmune-mediated hair follicle

a Division of Dermatology, Department of Medicine, University of Toronto School of Medicine, Toronto, Ontario, Canada; b Mediprobe Research Inc., 645 Windermere Road, London, Ontario N5X 2P1, Canada; c Cosmetic Skin and Surgery Center, 333 Sylvan Avenue, Suite 207, Englewood Cliffs, NJ 07632, USA
* Corresponding author. Mediprobe Research Inc., 645 Windermere Road, London, Ontario N5X 2P1, Canada.
E-mail address: agupta@mediproberesearch.com

Dermatol Clin 39 (2021) 429–445
https://doi.org/10.1016/j.det.2021.04.001
0733-8635/21/© 2021 Elsevier Inc. All rights reserved.

destruction is thought to play a role. Treatment of AA is challenging, with moderately effective treatment options including corticosteroids, immunosuppressants, topical immunotherapy, and light therapy.[7] Newer treatments are being evaluated, such as interleukin (IL)-2 agonists, IL-17 inhibitors, JAK inhibitors, platelet-rich plasma (PRP), and cell-based therapies.

Scarring alopecias often are a source of frustration for both physician and patient. In many forms of scarring alopecias, such as lichen planopilaris (LPP), the hair follicles are destroyed and a scar is formed, rendering conventional therapies useless. Treatments include topical corticosteroids, intralesional steroid injections, topical calcineurin inhibitor, oral corticosteroids, hydroxychloroquine, and immunosuppressive therapies; however, response rates to treatment are low.[8] PRP is an emerging therapy for LPP.

Regenerative medicine approaches to treating AGA and AA are gaining interest among physicians and patients and include PRP[9] and on the forefront of research, cell-based therapies. This article discusses the application and efficacy of these new therapies.

PLATELET-RICH PLASMA
History

One of the first uses of PRP in medicine was as an antihemorrhagic agent during cardiac surgery and for chronic nonhealing wounds.[10–12] Shortly thereafter, its regenerative properties on bone maturation and formation were exploited in dentistry.[13,14] The wound healing and tissue repair properties of PRP also began to be applied in areas, such as plastic surgery, orthopedics, and maxillofacial surgery.[15,16] In dermatology, PRP is used for scar revision, skin rejuvenation, wound healing, stretch marks, and hair restoration.[17–21] An attractive feature of PRP is that it is autologous; thus, the risk of immunogenic reactions and disease transmission between individuals is low.[22]

Preparation

PRP is a preparation of concentrated platelets found in plasma obtained by centrifugation of whole blood. Venous blood is collected from the patient into tubes containing an anticoagulant, either acid citrate dextrose or sodium citrate solution. The blood is centrifuged in order to separate it into 3 layers based on density (**Fig. 1**). The bottom layer contains red blood cells (RBCs) with leukocytes the middle layer is the PRP, and the top layer is platelet-poor plasma (PPP). The PPP is removed and the PRP is obtained for treatment. In some protocols, before injection into the scalp, PRP is activated by adding thrombin

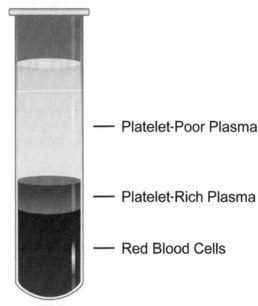

— Platelet-Poor Plasma

— Platelet-Rich Plasma

— Red Blood Cells

Fig. 1. Obtaining PRP from whole blood. Centrifugation separates whole blood into 3 layers: bottom, RBCs; middle, PRP; and top, PPP.

or calcium chloride, which promotes degranulation of α-granules and the release of growth factors.[23] There is no consensus as to whether platelets must be activated exogenously in order for PRP to exert its therapeutic effect.

There is a wide variety of protocols used to attain PRP that differ in centrifugation force, number and length of centrifugation cycles (single spin vs double spin), type of collection tubes, and whether an activation method was employed. This lends to differences in PRP composition across studies and could explain the large variability in the clinical benefit of PRP reported in the literature. It remains to be determined what the optimal PRP preparation method is for treating hair loss. One head-to-head trial compared 2 regimens of PRP treatments in patients with AGA.[24] One treatment group received 3 monthly treatments with a booster 3 months later; the other treatment group received 2 PRP treatments spaced 3 months apart. Assessment at 6 months found significant hair growth in both groups compared with baseline; however, the group with 3 monthly treatments also had significantly increased hair counts at 3 months, overall greater absolute and percentage change from baseline, and higher satisfaction scores compared with the group who received only 2 sessions of PRP spaced 3 months apart. Thus, this evidence suggests that monthly treatments of PRP may provide earlier and more profound hair growth; however, more studies are needed to confirm whether this regimen is ideal.

The normal range of circulating platelet levels is 150,000/μL to 400,000/μL in the blood.[25] The optimal concentration of platelets for the stimulation of angiogenesis has been shown to be 1.5 platelets/μL $\times$ 10^6 platelets/μL,[26] or 3 times to 10 times the concentration in whole blood. Some studies suggest that there is an optimal window of platelet concentration where the maximal effect is achieved, with higher concentrations having a paradoxically inhibitory effect.[27–29] Currently, however, there are no studies in humans that compare results of different concentrations of PRP on hair growth.

In an attempt to provide a step toward standardization of PRP preparations, the dose, efficiency, purity, and activation (DEPA) classification system has been proposed as a tool to determine the clinical impact of the variability of PRP compositions and to assess quality of PRP production.[30] PRP preparations reported using the DEPA classification will aid in comparing results across studies to determine the optimal PRP preparation method, optimal platelet concentration, and whether the addition of activators or presence of other cells is beneficial. Using the DEPA tool, the following data would be reported: dose of injected platelets, efficiency of production, purity of PRP obtained, and activation of PRP. The calculation of these parameters is possible only if complete cell counts are performed and volumes noted for both whole blood and PRP collected. The dose of injected platelets lends to approximating the dose of growth factors delivered to each injection site and is calculated by multiplying PRP platelet concentration by PRP volume. The efficiency of production of PRP heavily depends on the device used and is reported as percentage of platelets collected from whole blood. Purity of PRP is a measure of the relative composition of platelets, leukocytes, and RBCs. A pure preparation is deemed when the percentage of platelets compared with RBCs and leukocytes is greater than 90%. Some preparations are deemed leukocyte-poor, containing less leukocytes than whole blood, or leukocyte-rich (L-PRP), containing more leukocytes than whole blood. Whether or not the presence of leukocytes in PRP affects hair growth is not well understood. The final category in the DEPA classification is reporting the addition or absence of any exogenous activator, such as thrombin or calcium chloride. Ultimately, characterizing and reporting the type of PRP used will lead to a better understanding of the true effects of PRP as a treatment for hair loss.

Evidence of Platelet-Rich Plasma Efficacy for Treating Androgenetic Alopecia

Several randomized controlled trials (RCTs)[31–41] (**Table** 1) and numerous prospective cohort studies[24,42–56] have been published assessing PRP efficacy for AGA. There is considerable variability, however, in study design, PRP preparation method, treatment regimen, and quantification of outcomes, making it difficult to compare results across studies. Systematic reviews or meta-analyses of RCT data provide the highest level of evidence-based information; however, a lack of consistent outcomes across studies hinders the ability to perform these types of studies for PRP treatment for AGA. Outcomes vary from evaluation of clinical photographs and patient satisfaction surveys to hair density, hair diameter, and anagen-to-telogen ratios. Standardization of study outcomes in trials evaluating PRP for treatment of AGA is needed.

Parameters, such as hair density and diameter, are outcomes that can be compared across studies to estimate the true effect of PRP on hair growth. Taken together, data from studies evaluating these parameters suggest that PRP is efficacious in treating AGA, especially in men. Several studies have demonstrated that PRP significantly increases hair density in men,[20,21,31,33,38,40,42,54,57–59] with limited evidence available to draw strong conclusions for women.[20,21] It has been suggested that male patients and female patients should be investigated separately because PRP may have gender-specific effects and AGA in women is a multifactorial diseasae.[20,21] PRP has been reported to increase hair diameter in both genders,[21,35,42,54,57,60] although more studies are needed to confirm this effect.

A few studies have failed to show efficacy of PRP for treatment of AGA.[36,37,61] A double-blind, placebo-controlled pilot study investigating PRP for treatment of AGA in women found no effect on hair count or hair mass index 26 weeks after a single injection.[36] The ineffectiveness was attributed to inadequate frequency of injections, dilution of PRP with PPP, and no addition of an activating substance. A small, uncontrolled study investigating 5 injections of PRP every 2 weeks in 15 male patients with AGA failed to show any benefit from PRP 5 months after the initial injection.[61] Limitations of this study included low PRP platelet concentration (1.6-fold more than whole blood), small sample size, and low volume of PRP injected in each session. Lastly, a pilot RCT of 19 men did not find a significant effect of PRP for treatment of male AGA. Each patient was given 2 sessions of PRP or saline 1 month apart and numbers of terminal and vellus hairs assessed at 1 month, 3 months, and 6 months after the first injection.[37] Treatment failure in this study was attributed to patients having advanced hair loss (IV–VI on the Hamilton-Norwood scale) and of long duration of AGA (9 patients with 5–10 years' duration and 7

Table 1
Randomized controlled studies evaluating platelet-rich plasma efficacy for treatment of androgenetic alopecia

Study Identification No. of Participants	Platelet-rich Plasma Preparation	Treatment Regimen	Quantifiable Outcomes
Alves & Grimalt,[34] 2016 n = 25 (13 F, 12 M) Half-head study	• Centrifugations: single spin • Activator: calcium chloride • Platelet count: 3-fold increase from whole blood	PRP: 3 monthly PRP injections on half the scalp Control: saline injections into the contralateral scalp	3 mo and 6 mo: PRP significantly increased hair density compared with control areas only in the male participants.
Cervelli et al,[32] 2014 n = 10 M Half-head study	• Centrifugations: single spin • Activator: Ca^{2+} • Platelet count: 1.48 μL $\times 10^6$/μL	PRP: 3 monthly PRP injections into half the scalp Control: saline injections into the contralateral scalp	3 mo: PRP significantly increased hair density compared with control areas.
Dicle et al,[39] 2020 n = 15 M (first half of crossover trial)	• Centrifugations: single spin • Activator: physically activated with a bio-activator tube • Platelet count: not reported	PRP (10): 3 monthly PRP injections Control (15): 3 monthly saline injections	4 mo: no statistically significant difference between hair densities after injections of PRP vs injections of placebo
Dubin et al,[41] 2020 n = 30 F	• Centrifugations: single spin • Activator: none • Platelet count: not reported	PRP (15): 3 monthly PRP injections Control (15): 3 monthly saline injections	2 mo and 6 mo: PRP significantly increased hair density compared with placebo 6 mo: PRP significantly increased hair caliber compared with placebo.
Gentile,[31] 2015 n = 23 M Half-head study	• Centrifugations: single spin • Activator: Ca^{2+} • Platelet count: 1.48 μL $\times 10^6$/μL	PRP: 3 monthly PRP injection into half the scalp Control: saline injections into the contralateral scalp	3 mo: PRP significantly increased hair density and terminal hair density compared with control areas.
Gentile et al,[33] 2017 n = 18 M Half-head study	• Centrifugations: single spin • Activator: none • Platelet count: not reported	PRP: 3 monthly PRP injection into half the scalp Control: saline injections into the contralateral scalp	3 mo: PRP significantly increased hair density compared with control areas.
Mapar et al,[37] 2016 n = 19 M Half-head study	• Centrifugations: double spin • Activator: calcium gluconate • Platelet count: 3-fold increase from whole blood	Two 2.5-cm × 2.5-cm square areas on each patient were randomly assigned either: PRP: 2 monthly PRP injections into a 2.5-cm × 2.5-cm square area Control: 2 monthly saline injections into a 2.5-cm × 2.5-cm square area	6 mo: PRP did not significantly change terminal or vellus hair counts compared with control areas.

(continued on next page)

Table 1
(continued)

Study Identification No. of Participants	Platelet-rich Plasma Preparation	Treatment Regimen	Quantifiable Outcomes
Puig et al,[36] 2016 n = 26 F	• Centrifugations: single spin • Activator: none • Platelet count: 2.75-fold–3.4-fold increase from whole blood	PRP (15): single session of injections of PRP Control (11): single session of injections of saline	6 mo: PRP had no significant effect on hair density or caliber.
Rodrigues et al,[38] 2019 n = 26 M	• Centrifugations: double spin • Activator: autologous serum • Platelet count: 1200/µL × 10^6/µL	PRP (15): 4 sessions of PRP injections spaced 15 d apart Control (11): 4 sessions of saline injections spaced 15 d apart	3 mo: PRP significantly increased hair density and percent anagen hairs compared with control group.
Singh et al,[40] 2020 n = 80 M	• Centrifugation: double spin • Activator: calcium gluconate • Platelet count: 4.2-fold higher than whole blood	Topical minoxidil (20): minoxidil 5% twice daily + 3 monthly intradermal saline injections, for 3 mo PRP + minoxidil (20): minoxidil 5% twice daily + 3 monthly intradermal PRP injections, for 3 mo Placebo (20): topical placebo twice daily + 3 monthly intradermal saline injections, for 3 mo PRP (20): topical placebo twice daily + 3 monthly intradermal PRP injections, for 3 mo	5 mo: all 3 treatment groups significantly increased hair density compared with the placebo group. The maximum improvement was found in the PRP + minoxidil group followed by PRP monotherapy, then minoxidil monotherapy. A decrease in hair density was found in the placebo group.
Tawfik and Osman,[35] 2018 n = 30 F Half-head study	• Centrifugation: double spin • Activator: calcium gluconate • Platelet count: not reported	PRP: 4 weekly PRP injections into select area of scalp Control: 4 weekly saline injections into another region of the scalp	6.75 mo: PRP significantly increased hair density and caliber compared with control areas.

Abbreviations: F, female; M, male; n, number of participants; mo, month; Ca2+, Calcium2+.

patients with >10 years' duration). Overall, inadequate response to PRP in these studies was attributed to low number and frequency of injections, inadequate platelet concentration, high severity of AGA in the patient population, and/or long duration of baldness of the patients.

A variety of PRP combinations have been tested in an effort to improve efficacy. PRP has been combined with suture embedding and microneedling with successful results[62,63] as well as with dalteparin and protamine microparticles.[64] These microparticles are carriers for controlled release of growth factors. This study[64] found that both PRP monotherapy and PRP in combination with microparticles enhanced hair growth, but the combination facilitated greater hair growth compared with PRP monotherapy. In another study, a significant increase in mean hair number and thickness was observed in patients 3 months and 6 months after injections of PRP supplemented with CD34$^+$ cells (known to have angiogenic effects); however, whether this effect is greater than PRP alone is not known because no comparison group was assessed.[65] Another formulation of PRP used for treatment of hair loss in a few case studies with successful results is a gel-like product referred to as plasma-rich fibrin.[66–68] Additionally, several practitioners offer patients treatment of hair loss using a combination of PRP with ACell technology in the United States. ACell is a regenerative medicine product used to heal wounds by acting like a scaffold for new tissue growth and promotes angiogenesis and tissue healing.[69] Many clinics offer this combination and report successful results; however, no clinical trials have been published.

A few studies have assessed PRP in combination with minoxidil. One study of male patients with AGA found that combination PRP plus minoxidil 5% solution significantly increased hair density and diameter and decreased the proportion of telogen hairs compared with PRP or minoxidil 5% solution alone.[70] A half-head study assessed the effect of PRP or placebo in patients on either topical minoxidil 5% solution twice daily or finasteride, 1 mg per day.[71] Compared with placebo, PRP significantly increased hair density in patients on either minoxidil or finasteride. PRP combined with minoxidil resulted in significantly increased hair density, percentage of anagen hair, and anagen-to-telogen ratio compared with PRP in combination with finasteride.

PRP also has been combined with stromal vascular fraction (SVF) from adipose tissue to successfully induce hair growth in patients with AGA.[72] The resulting combination was platelet-rich stroma (PRS). SVF contains adipose-derived stromal cells (mesenchymal stem cells) as well as hematopoietic stem and progenitor cells, endothelial cells, erythrocytes, fibroblasts, lymphocytes, monocytes/macrophages, and pericytes.[73] Ten male patients with AGA (Hamilton-Norwood IIa–VII) received a single session of PRS (5 mL PRP + 1 mL SVF, mixed). A significant increase in hair density was found at 6 weeks and 12 weeks after the injection. This study also reported the observation of PRS-induced regrowth of hair shafts from yellow dots (empty follicles filled with sebum or keratitic material).[72] No side effects were noted. Because a significant increase in hair density was detected after a single injection, this study suggests that the combination of PRP with SVF may be more effective than PRP alone. Additional studies are needed to confirm this effect and compare the efficacy of PRS to PRP monotherapy.

Standardization of the number of treatments, frequency of treatments, and whether a booster is needed to maintain any positive effects is lacking. Currently, most evidence supports 3 sessions of PRP at 1-month intervals followed by a maintenance regimen.[20] More studies comparing treatment regimens are needed, however, to confirm this finding.

Based on findings reported in the literature and the authors' own experiences and successes (**Fig. 2**), the authors recommend 2-times to 4-times platelet concentration, minimizing RBCs and white blood cells, and subdermal injections of 3 sessions to 4 sessions of PRP at 1-month intervals followed by a maintenance regimen of 2 times to 4 times per year, depending on results. The authors also recommend 0.3-mL to 0.5-mL injection volume, depending on volume of PRP obtained, and 1-cm to 2.5-cm space between injections in the affected area, again depending on the volume of PRP.

Evidence of Platelet-Rich Plasma Efficacy for Treating Alopecia Areata

AA has an unpredictable course, with 34% to 50% of patients recovering within 1 year and 14% to 25% of patients progressing to alopecia totalis or alopecia universalis.[74] Evidence regarding the effectiveness of PRP for treatment of AA is preliminary, but promising.[75]

Two RCTs have shown significant improvement of hair growth in localized AA patients after PRP treatment.[76,77] One study found that 3 sessions of PRP every month significantly increased hair growth in male patients and female patients up to 12 months after the initial injection compared with placebo and intralesional triamcinolone (2.5 mg/cm^3).[77] The second study treated patients with 3 treatments of PRP spaced monthly, placebo (topical panthenol cream) applied twice daily, or minoxidil 5% applied twice daily and found both PRP and minoxidil to increase hair growth significantly compared with the control group at 3 months after the initial treatment.[76] PRP also significantly decreased short vellus hairs, yellow dots, and dystrophic hair whereas minoxidil did not.

PRP also has improved hair regrowth in patients with AA in 2 nonrandomized trials.[78,79] One study treated patients with intralesional injections of either triamcinolone (10 mg/mL) or 3 sessions of PRP at 3-week intervals.[78] The overall improvement at the end of 9 weeks was 100% for all patients in both treatment groups. This study concluded that PRP was efficacious and safe for treating AA with efficacy comparable to triamcinolone. A prospective study conducted in 20 patients with AA found that 6 sessions of PRP at monthly intervals promoted good hair growth in all but 1 patient at 6 months and 1-year post-treatment.[79] No quantifiable outcome, however, was assessed in this study. No serious side effects were reported in either study.

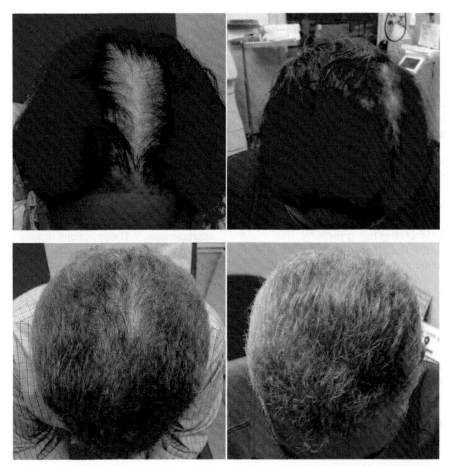

Fig. 2. Before and after photographic examples of PRP treatment of AGA. (*Top*) A 38-year-old woman before (*left*) and after (*right*) 7 treatments of PRP. This patient also was taking finasteride. (*Bottom*) A48-year-old man before (*left*) and after (*right*) 5 sessions of PRP. Photographs courtesy of Jeffrey Rapaport, MD.

Two case reports support the positive effect of PRP for AA[80,81]; however, a case series of 9 patients found only limited efficacy of PRP for treating chronic (>2 years), severe (>50% involvement) alopecia areata.[82] In this case series, patients received 3 sessions of PRP at 45-day to 60-day intervals. The platelet concentration was approximately 3-fold to 4-fold higher than whole blood, and the PRP was activated with calcium gluconate. At 8 months, 6 subjects showed regrowth of terminal pigmented hair with the other patients noting nonpigmented vellus hair growth; however, assessment at 1 year revealed that none of the patients retained the new hair growth. This study suggests that PRP does not provide persistent results and failed to prevent relapses in severe forms of AA; however, larger studies are required to confirm this finding.

Overall, although limited, there is evidence to support the use of PRP for treatment, especially in mild to moderate localized AA, and it seems

relatively safe. The number of PRP sessions required and optimal PRP preparation method have yet to be standardized, precluding any recommendations. Larger-scale, RCTs are needed to confirm the efficacy of PRP for AA and evaluate where it fits into the arsenal of treatment options.

Evidence of platelet-rich plasma efficacy for treating lichen planopilaris

LPP is classified as a primary lymphocytic scarring alopecia whose treatment remains a challenge and cause is unknown. One of the first reports of the use of PRP for LPP was a case report of a patient with LPP who failed previous treatments. The patient was administered PRP therapy in 3 sessions and experienced complete regression of itching and hair shedding when evaluated at the 6 month follow-up appointment.[83] Another case study treated a patient with LPP with a combination of topical minoxidil 2% with 4 sessions of PRP 3 weeks apart and observed hair thickening, concluding that PRP could be an effective adjunctive treatment of LPP.[84] These case reports are promising, warranting larger trials of evaluating the efficacy of PRP for treatment of LPP.

Mechanism of Action

Platelets were once thought to function only as hemostatic regulators; however, recent research has shed light on the possible new roles of platelets in inflammation, angiogenesis, stem cell migration, and cell proliferation through the release of growth factors and cytokines.[25,85,86] Growth factors released from α granules of platelets in PRP are believed to be key mediators in the mechanisms involved in stimulating hair growth.[23]

Evidence suggests that the etiology of AGA, in part, is mediated by dihydrotestosterone (DHT) inhibition of growth factor signaling, leading to hair follicle miniaturization.[87,88] For example, in mice, DHT inhibits hair growth through the inhibition of insulinlike growth factor 1 (IGF-1) signaling.[87] An innovative source of IGF-1, as well as other growth factors that promote hair regrowth, is PRP. It is thought that these growth factors promote cell proliferation, differentiation, angiogenesis, and chemotaxis necessary for hair regrowth.[23,89,90]

Growth factors reported in high concentrations in PRP include IGF-1, platelet-derived growth factor, transforming growth factor (TGF)-β, vascular endothelial growth factor (VEGF), epidermal growth factor (EGF), fibroblast growth factor (FGF),[91(p)119] and glial cell line–derived neurotrophic factor (GDNF).[92] Many of these growth factors have been shown to foster vascularization, increasing the supply of nutrients and oxygen to the follicle to support hair growth.[64,93,94] This mechanism is thought to counteract the reduced blood flow and oxygen pressure detected in AGA.[95]

The range in growth factor concentrations in PRP can vary greatly across individuals and preparation methods,[92] which may contribute to the variation in reports on PRP efficacy. Growth factors in PRP found to correlate with increased hair density in treated patients include GDNF and VEGF.[92] The direct effect of GDNF on hair growth is unknown; however, GDNF and its receptors are expressed in hair follicle cells, and there is evidence that suggests this growth factor promotes cell proliferation and protects from premature catagen transition.[96–99] The role of VEGF in hair growth is more clear because this factor is known to be a potent hair growth stimulant, likely through induction of angiogenesis.[100,101] Possible toxicities associated with higher concentrations of VEGF, however, have been reported in other areas of medicine, such as diseases of the central nervous system,[102–104] and there are negative side effects associated with certain growth factors approved for therapy.[105] Thus, it is possible that PRP containing high concentrations of certain growth factors could have a negative impact on hair growth. This lends more evidence to the theory that there is a therapeutic window for PRP where optimal growth factor concentrations promote maximal hair growth but outside of this window can have no effect or even be detrimental.

Lastly, there is evidence suggesting growth factors stimulate telogen to anagen transition and can extend the length of anagen by preventing apoptosis as well as induce vascularization and angiogenesis.[27] These actions require growth factors to bind to their corresponding cellular receptor(s) to initiate downstream signaling, ultimately affecting gene expression of factors that promote hair growth.[106(p2)] Two pathways are thought to play key roles: extracellular signal-regulated kinase and protein kinase B.[27] Ultimately, the activation of these pathways promotes faster telogen to anagen transition,[27] preventing apoptosis and facilitating cell growth and prolonged survival of hair follicles.[27(p2),64]

CELL-BASED THERAPY
History

There is great enthusiasm over the therapeutic potential of stems cells and their products. Stem cells often are considered the next frontier of medicine and promise to yield treatments for previously incurable diseases. Although the progress of stem cell therapies has been slower than anticipated, applications are being realized in many fields, including hair restoration.

Stem cells are defined by their ability to both self-renew and differentiate into other cellular subtypes. In 1998, researchers from the University of Wisconsin published a groundbreaking article describing derivation and culture of human embryonic stem cells,[107] generating excitement over the potential advancement of drug discovery and transplantation medicine. The many ethical and political issues that accompanied the use of human embryonic stem cells, however, hampered research progress. In pursuit of an alternative, research into the potential therapeutic use of adult stems cells was ignited.

Adult stem cells from the bone marrow were among the first to be discovered and used therapeutically.[108] It is now known that adult multipotent stem cells are present in far more tissues and organs than once thought, such as skin, liver, digestive epithelium, dental pulp, hair follicles, and adipose tissue. The discovery that adipose tissue harbors stem cells was published in 2002[109] and introduced a convenient and accessible means to harvest adult stem cells for therapeutic uses, paving a new path for regenerative medicine exploration. Since then, adipose stem cells have been exploited in many areas of medicinal research,[110] including their recent application as a treatment of hair loss.[111]

The benefits of stem cells may not be restricted to the cell itself, with more recent evidence suggesting a role for their secreted factors,[112] such as exosomes.[113] The potential therapeutic effect of exosomes recently has generated excitement in the field of hair restoration with some clinics offering this therapy and reporting impressive results; however, research still is in preliminary level and whether exosomes will be a game-changer in hair restoration remains to be determined.

Mechanism of action

The hair follicle is a regenerating miniorgan, which undergoes cycles of growth (anagen), regression (catagen), and rest (telogen). Hair follicle stem cells and their paracrine signaling play a critical role in regulating hair cycling.[114] Stem cell niches within the hair follicle reside in the bulge region, dermal papilla, and hair germ. The transition from telogen to anagen is initiated by signaling from cells in the hair germ. Subsequently, stem cells in the bulge region and dermal papilla begin to proliferate and differentiate, resulting in the production of a new, terminal hair shaft. The molecular mechanisms that modulate stem cell activity, and thus hair follicle cycling, remain elusive, but a few key players have been identified.[114]

Critical regulators of stem cell quiescence, proliferation, and differentiation during hair follicle cycling include Wnt, bone morphogenetic protein (BMP), and FGF18.[115–118] Stem cells in the dermal papilla and bulge region are maintained in a quiescent state during telogen via BMP, TGF-β, FGF, and Wnt inhibitor signaling.[118–122] Anagen phase can be stimulated by activation of Wnt signaling and β-catenin.[114,118,123,124]

It generally is accepted that follicle miniaturization exhibited in AGA is driven by androgens. There is evidence that androgens deregulate dermal papilla cell paracrine signaling by inhibiting the Wnt signaling pathway.[125] Thus, it is speculated that cell-based therapies for AGA promote hair growth by providing the signals needed to reinstate or initiate dermal papilla cell cross talk, stimulating this cell population to proliferate and differentiate, pushing the follicle into anagen phase.

Applications in Hair Loss

Cell-based therapies, although newer in their application in hair restoration, show promising results for the effective treatment of AGA and AA. There are several different preparations of cell-based therapies that have been utilized for treatment of hair loss that include adipose-derived stromal cells, stem cells obtained from hair follicles, adipose tissue–derived stem cell conditioned media (ADSC-CM), autologous bone marrow–derived mononuclear cells, autologous follicular stem cells, and exosomes. A novel stem cell educator therapy also has been tested.

Studies Investigating Cell-based Therapies for Androgenetic Alopecia

Adipose-derived stem cell constituent

There has been 1 randomized, placebo-controlled study conducted to determine the efficacy and safety of topically applied adipose-derived stem cell constituent (ADSC-CE) for treatment of AGA.[111] ADSC-CE was prepared by enzymatically isolating stem cells from healthy donor adipose tissue and then cultured in vitro. One million cells were resuspended in distilled water and cell membranes disrupted by low-frequency ultrasound. The test solution was diluted to 1% ADSC-CE with distilled water and patients applied 2 mL twice daily to hair loss areas for 16 weeks. Patients in the placebo group applied distilled water in the same regimen. A significant increase in hair density was observed at 8 weeks and 16 weeks after initial treatment in the ADSC-CE treated group compared with the placebo group. A significant increase in hair diameter was detected at 16 weeks in the ADSC-CE treated group. ADSC-CE was well tolerated and no major adverse effects were noted. This study was conducted in a small population (n = 19 in each group) and, despite randomization, the ADSC-CE treated group had significantly lower hair count at baseline compared with the control group.[111]

Adipose tissue–derived stem cell conditioned media

ADSC-CM generally is attained by enzymatically digesting adipose tissue obtained by medical liposuction to collect the stromal cell fraction, which then is filtered. ADSCs obtained by this process are cultured and the conditioned media collected and used as treatment, under the theory that secreted factors carry out stem cell functions. There is evidence supporting that the secretome of adipose-derived stem cells, including cytokines and exosomes, provides a beneficial paracrine effect on the surrounding cells and tissues.[126–128]

A few studies have investigated the effects of ADSC-CM on hair growth in patients with AGA. A retrospective, observational study of 27 female patients with Ludwig type I AGA evaluated the efficacy of ADSC-CM applied once a week via microneedling for 12 weeks.[129] At 12 weeks, hair density and diameter significantly increased compared with baseline. Other studies have also shown a positive effect of ADSC-CM on hair growth. Six injections of ADSC-CM at 3-week to 5-week intervals significantly increased hair counts in male patients (n = 11) and female patients (n = 11) with alopecia; however, the type of alopecia was not specified.[130,131] A prospective study on 40 male patients and female patients with AGA evaluated 6 intradermal injections of ADSC-CM spaced monthly and reported that, compared with baseline, this treatment significantly improved hair density and anagen rate, but terminal hair density did not change.[132]

Adipose tissue–derived stromal vascular fraction and adipose-derived stem cells

SVF is a heterogenous cell population consisting of circulating blood cells, fibroblasts, pericytes, and endothelial cells as well as adipocyte stem cells.[133] Conversely, ASCs are a more homogenous cell population consisting of isolated, plastic-adherent, multipotent stem cell.

A study of 9 patients employed scalp injections of SVF for treatment of AGA and found the treatment significantly increased hair density but not anagen percentage, telogen percentage, or cumulative thickness at 24 weeks after treatment.[134] The study also found that this procedure was safe and well tolerated in patients with AGA. One patient suffered a hematoma in the region of the hairline during the injection of SVF, which was self-limiting and did not require any intervention other than observation. Although this study shows promising results for use of SVF for AGA, it has limitations, including open-label, nonblinded analysis, and small sample size; thus, larger studies are needed to confirm this effect.

A prospective, randomized, multicenter trial tested the clinical effectiveness of injections of adipose-derived regenerative cell-enriched (ADRC) purified fat for the treatment of AGA in 71 (17 female and 54 male) patients.[135] Lipoaspirate was prepared at 2 different cell concentrations to test whether cell concentration affected the outcome. There were no statistically significant changes in total hair count or hair width between the low-dose ADRC, high-dose ADRC, or fat-alone control groups and the no-fat saline control group at any timepoint. When an ad hoc subgroup of male patients with Hamilton-Norwood III was analyzed, however, the low-dose ADRC treatment significantly increased hair counts and hair width at 6 weeks, 12 weeks, and 24 weeks compared with baseline. Additionally, low-dose ADRC treatment significantly increased hair count in this subgroup compared with no-fat saline control at 24 weeks. The effects were not maintained, however, at 1 year. The procedure was well tolerated and no adverse events were reported. The investigators conclude that this approach is promising and warrants further research for treatment of early patterned hair loss.

As discussed previously, a study investigating the synergistic effects of adipose-derived stromal cells combined with PRP for treatment of AGA found that this treatment significantly induced hair growth.[72]

Stem cells from human hair follicles

Stem cells have been isolated from human hair follicle punch biopsies and used to treat 11 patients with AGA.[136] This novel approach used centrifugation instead of culture conditions to isolate stem cells. Scalp tissue was excised via punch biopsy and excess adipose tissue removed. Tissue was disaggregated with the use of a medical device (Rigeneracons®, based on Rigenera protocol, Italy) and then centrifuged. The cell suspension then was collected and administered as interfollicular injections at a depth of 5 mm. Each patient was treated with 2 sessions spaced 60 days apart; 23 weeks after the last treatment, mean hair density was reported to have increased 29% over baseline in the stem cell–treated group compared with only 1% in the placebo group. No statistics were reported; thus, it is difficult to make conclusions from these results, but they do provide intrigue into this method that warrants further investigation.

Mesenchymal stem cell–derived exosomes

Exosomes are extracellular vesicles that relay signaling molecules, such as transcription factors, cytokines, and microRNA, from 1 cell to another. Dermal papilla cell–derived exosomes have been deemed important modulators of paracrine signaling involved in hair follicle regeneration.[137] Exosome treatment of hair loss is a field that is rapidly gaining momentum as anecdotal reports of successful exosome therapy for hair loss are surfacing. Although there are preclinical studies (in vitro and animal studies) that show favorable outcomes of exosome treatment-induced hair growth, there currently are no published clinical studies testing the efficacy of exosome therapy for hair growth in humans.[113] Presentations from innovators at the International Society of Hair Restoration Surgeons (ISHRS) World Congress in 2020 showed promising preliminary results from ongoing trials of exosome treatment o AA[138] and AGA.[139] Currently, there are 8 different exosome companies producing exosomes from various sources.

Exosomes are an exciting prospective treatment because many clinicians who employ this treatment report marked hair growth that is visible much earlier than that from any other treatment (PRP, minoxidil, and finasteride). This treatment remains in its infancy, however, data from large clinical trials are needed to determine efficacy. Additionally, the FDA issued a warning regarding the application of exosomes for therapy of any kind. The warning states that there currently are no FDA-approved exosome products and is intended to inform the public of multiple recent reports of serious adverse events experienced by patients in Nebraska following exosome therapy.[140]

Studies Investigating Cell-based Therapies for Alopecia Areata

Adipose-derived stromal vascular cells
One retrospective study has tested adipose-derived stromal vascular cells (ADSVCs), obtained via lipoaspirate, as a treatment of AA in 20 patients.[141] To isolate ADSVC, lipoaspirate was centrifuged to remove debris and RBCs and then enzyme digested. After a series of centrifugation and filtering, the SVF was collected and number of viable cells determined. The treatment was injected into balding areas of the scalp at a depth of 4 mm, 0.2 mL per injection, spaced 1 cm apart. A total of 5 mL was injected into 25 sites. Hair density and diameter significantly increased at 3 months and 6 months after treatment compared with untreated controls.[141]

Stem cell educator method
A novel method, termed *stem cell educator therapy*, was tested in an open label, phase I/II study for treatment of severe AA in 9 patients.[142] With this technique, the patient's blood is circulated through a system that separates mononuclear cells from whole blood. These separated cells then interact with adherent human cord blood–derived multipotent stem cells, which are thought to modulate or reprogram monocytes to restore immune tolerance. These now educated mononuclear cells return to a patient's circulation and are thought to bestow immune balance and homeostasis within the patients. All but 1 patient in the study experienced improved hair regrowth in varying degrees at 12 weeks post-treatment.[142]

Bone marrow–derived mononuclear cells and follicular stem cells
In a randomized study of 40 patients (20 with AGA and 20 with AA), patients were treated with either autologous bone marrow–derived mononuclear cells, or autologous follicular stem cells.[143] Mononuclear cells were isolated from bone marrow harvested from the upper iliac crest through a series of filtrations and centrifugations. Follicular stem cells were obtained and cultured from a 4-mm skin punch biopsy from an unaffected area of the scalp. Intradermal injections of the treatments were performed per square centimeter of the balding area. Both AA and AGA showed significant improvement in hair density and diameter 6 months after a single injection of either therapy, with no difference between the 2 types of stem cell treatment.[143]

SUMMARY

Regenerative medicine approaches for treatment of AGA and AA are promising; however, further RCTs with large sample sizes and longer follow-up periods are needed to confirm the reported efficacies. PRP appears to be safe because no serious adverse events have been reported and side effects appear to be minimal. Evaluation of cell-based therapies for efficacy and safety is needed. There is a need for standardization of treatment preparation as well as treatment regimen, including dose, number, and interval of treatment sessions, and injection technique. For PRP, most reports support monthly injections of at least 3 months. Additionally, the outcomes reported in studies vary considerably, making cross-study comparisons difficult. The authors recommend studies to include the quantifiable outcomes of hair density, hair diameter, and anagen-to-telogen ratios to aid comparisons and the combining of results to determine clinical efficacy.

CLINICS CARE POINTS

Pearls

- A complete hair consultation is necessary to determine proper therapy.

- There is a variation in the protocols reported for obtaining Platelet Rich Plasma (PRP): for example, Double spin centrifugation vs Single spin centrifugation; nonetheless, mechanical agitation is recommended to separate platelets from the gel tubes.

- Adequate platelet count is important prior to initiating PRP therapy (greater than 105,000).
- Combination therapy of PRP with other therapeutic interventions has demonstrated superior efficacy compared to monotherapy.
- Treatment in patients with an early onset or a shorter duration of hair loss usually leads to better results.

Pitfalls

- Treatment course and patient expectation may not align with the prognosis as hair loss is a multi-factorial condition.

DISCLOSURE

A.K. Gupta, H.J. Renaud, and J.A. Rapaport have no financial interests or conflicts of interest to declare. No grants or sponsorships were received to support this article.

REFERENCES

1. Tabolli S, Sampogna F, di Pietro C, et al. Health status, coping strategies, and alexithymia in subjects with androgenetic alopecia: a questionnaire study. Am J Clin Dermatol 2013;14(2):139–45.
2. Santos Z, Avci P, Hamblin MR. Drug discovery for alopecia: gone today, hair tomorrow. Expert Opin Drug Discov 2015;10(3):269–92.
3. Lolli F, Pallotti F, Rossi A, et al. Androgenetic alopecia: a review. Endocrine 2017;57(1):9–17.
4. Gupta AK, Foley KA. A critical assessment of the evidence for low-level laser therapy in the treatment of hair loss. Dermatol Surg 2017;43(2): 188–97.
5. Gupta AK, Mays RR, Dotzert MS, et al. Efficacy of non-surgical treatments for androgenetic alopecia: a systematic review and network meta-analysis. J Eur Acad Dermatol Venereol 2018;32(12):2112–25.
6. Mirzoyev SA, Schrum AG, Davis MDP, et al. Lifetime Incidence Risk of Alopecia Areata Estimated at 2.1% by Rochester Epidemiology Project, 1990–2009. J Invest Dermatol 2014;134(4):1141–2.
7. Pratt CH, King LE, Messenger AG, et al. Alopecia areata. Nat Rev Dis Primer 2017;3:17011.
8. Lyakhovitsky A, Amichai B, Sizopoulou C, et al. A case series of 46 patients with lichen planopilaris: Demographics, clinical evaluation, and treatment experience. J Dermatol Treat 2015;26(3): 275–9.
9. Gupta AK, Quinlan EM. Changing Trends in Surgical Hair Restoration: Use of Google Trends and the ISHRS Practice Census Survey. J Cosmet Dermatol 2020;19(11):2974–81.
10. Cieslik-Bielecka A, Choukroun J, Odin G, et al. L-PRP/L-PRF in esthetic plastic surgery, regenerative medicine of the skin and chronic wounds. Curr Pharm Biotechnol 2012;13(7):1266–77.
11. Ferrari M, Zia S, Valbonesi M, et al. A new technique for hemodilution, preparation of autologous platelet-rich plasma and intraoperative blood salvage in cardiac surgery. Int J Artif Organs 1987;10(1):47–50.
12. DelRossi AJ, Cernaianu AC, Vertrees RA, et al. Platelet-rich plasma reduces postoperative blood loss after cardiopulmonary bypass. J Thorac Cardiovasc Surg 1990;100(2):281–6.
13. Marx RE, Carlson ER, Eichstaedt RM, et al. Platelet-rich plasma: Growth factor enhancement for bone grafts. Oral Surg Oral Med Oral Pathol Oral Radiol Endod 1998;85(6):638–46.
14. Anitua E. Plasma rich in growth factors: preliminary results of use in the preparation of future sites for implants. Int J Oral Maxillofac Implants 1999; 14(4):529–35.
15. Albanese A, Licata ME, Polizzi B, et al. Platelet-rich plasma (PRP) in dental and oral surgery: from the wound healing to bone regeneration. Immun Ageing A 2013;10(1):23.
16. Nguyen RT, Borg-Stein J, McInnis K. Applications of platelet-rich plasma in musculoskeletal and sports medicine: an evidence-based approach. PM R 2011;3(3):226–50.
17. Lin M-Y, Lin C-S, Hu S, et al. Progress in the Use of Platelet-rich Plasma in Aesthetic and Medical Dermatology. J Clin Aesthet Dermatol 2020;13(8): 28–35.
18. Gupta AK, Carviel JL. Meta-analysis of efficacy of platelet-rich plasma therapy for androgenetic alopecia. J Dermatol Treat 2017;28(1):55–8.
19. Gupta AK, Versteeg SG, Rapaport J, et al. The Efficacy of Platelet-Rich Plasma in the Field of Hair Restoration and Facial Aesthetics-A Systematic Review and Meta-analysis. J Cutan Med Surg 2019. https://doi.org/10.1177/1203475418818073.
20. Gupta AK, Cole J, Deutsch DP, et al. Platelet-Rich Plasma as a Treatment for Androgenetic Alopecia. Dermatol Surg 2019;45(10):1262–73. https://doi.org/10.1097/DSS.0000000000001894.
21. Gupta AK, Renaud HJ, Bamimore M. Platelet-rich plasma for androgenetic alopecia: Efficacy differences between men and women. Dermatol Ther 2020;e14143. https://doi.org/10.1111/dth.14143.
22. Arshdeep, Kumaran MS. Platelet-rich plasma in dermatology: boon or a bane? Indian J Dermatol Venereol Leprol 2014;80(1):5–14.
23. Gupta AK, Carviel J. A Mechanistic Model of Platelet-Rich Plasma Treatment for Androgenetic Alopecia. Dermatol Surg 2016;42(12):1335–9.
24. Hausauer A, Jones D. Evaluating the efficacy of different platelet-rich plasma regimens for

management of androgenetic alopecia: a single-center, blinded, randomized clinical trial. Dermatol Surg 2018;44(9):1191–200.

25. Alves R, Grimalt R. A review of platelet-rich plasma: history, biology, mechanism of action, and classification. Skin Appendage Disord 2018;4(1):18–24.

26. Giusti I, Rughetti A, D'Ascenzo S, et al. Identification of an optimal concentration of platelet gel for promoting angiogenesis in human endothelial cells. Transfusion (Paris) 2009;49(4):771–8.

27. Li ZJ, Choi H-I, Choi D-K, et al. Autologous platelet-rich plasma: a potential therapeutic tool for promoting hair growth. Dermatol Surg 2012;38(7 Pt 1):1040–6.

28. Graziani F, Ivanovski S, Cei S, et al. The in vitro effect of different PRP concentrations on osteoblasts and fibroblasts. Clin Oral Implants Res 2006;17(2):212–9.

29. Weibrich G, Hansen T, Kleis W, et al. Effect of platelet concentration in platelet-rich plasma on peri-implant bone regeneration. Bone 2004;34(4):665–71.

30. Magalon J, Chateau AL, Bertrand B, et al. DEPA classification: a proposal for standardising PRP use and a retrospective application of available devices. BMJ Open Sport Exerc Med 2016;2(1). https://doi.org/10.1136/bmjsem-2015-000060.

31. Gentile P, Garcovich S, Bielli A, et al. The effect of platelet-rich plasma in hair regrowth: a randomized placebo-controlled trial. Stem Cells Transl Med 2015;4(11):1317–23.

32. Cervelli V, Garcovich S, Bielli A, et al. The effect of autologous activated platelet rich plasma (AA-PRP) injection on pattern hair loss: clinical and histomorphometric evaluation. Biomed Res Int 2014;2014:760709.

33. Gentile P, Cole JP, Cole MA, et al. Evaluation of Not-Activated and Activated PRP in Hair Loss Treatment: Role of Growth Factor and Cytokine Concentrations Obtained by Different Collection Systems. Int J Mol Sci 2017;18(2). https://doi.org/10.3390/ijms18020408.

34. Alves R, Grimalt R. Randomized Placebo-Controlled, Double-Blind, Half-Head Study to Assess the Efficacy of Platelet-Rich Plasma on the Treatment of Androgenetic Alopecia. Dermatol Surg 2016;42(4):491–7.

35. Tawfik AA, Osman MAR. The effect of autologous activated platelet-rich plasma injection on female pattern hair loss: A randomized placebo-controlled study. J Cosmet Dermatol 2018;17:47–53.

36. Puig CJ, Reese R, Peters M. Double-blind, placebo-controlled pilot study on the use of platelet-rich plasma in women with female androgenetic alopecia. Dermatol Surg 2016;42(11):1243–7.

37. Mapar MA, Shahriari S, Haghighizadeh MH. Efficacy of platelet-rich plasma in the treatment of androgenetic (male-patterned) alopecia: A pilot randomized controlled trial. J Cosmet Laser Ther 2016;18(8):452–5.

38. Rodrigues BL, Montalvão SAL, Cancela RBB, et al. Treatment of male pattern alopecia with platelet-rich plasma: A double-blind controlled study with analysis of platelet number and growth factor levels. J Am Acad Dermatol 2019;80(3):694–700.

39. Dicle Ö, Bilgic Temel A, Gülkesen KH. Platelet-rich plasma injections in the treatment of male androgenetic alopecia: A randomized placebo-controlled crossover study. J Cosmet Dermatol 2020;19(5):1071–7.

40. Singh SK, Kumar V, Rai T. Comparison of efficacy of platelet-rich plasma therapy with or without topical 5% minoxidil in male-type baldness: A randomized, double-blind placebo control trial. Indian J Dermatol Venereol Leprol 2020;86(2):150–7.

41. Dubin DP, Lin MJ, Leight HM, et al. The effect of platelet-rich plasma on female androgenetic alopecia: a randomized controlled trial. J Am Acad Dermatol 2020. https://doi.org/10.1016/j.jaad.2020.06.1021.

42. Kapoor R, Shome D, Vadera S, et al. 678 & QR678 Neo Vs PRP-A randomised, comparative, prospective study. J Cosmet Dermatol 2020. https://doi.org/10.1111/jocd.13398.

43. Anitua E, Pino A, Martinez N, et al. The effect of plasma rich in growth factors on pattern hair loss: A pilot study. Dermatol Surg 2017;43(5):658–70.

44. Borhan R, Gasnier C, Reygagne P. Autologous Platelet Rich Plasma as a Treatment of Male Androgenetic Alopecia: Study of 14 Cases. J Clin Exp Dermatol Res 2015;6(4):1–6.

45. Butt G, Hussain I, Ahmed FJ, et al. Efficacy of platelet-rich plasma in androgenetic alopecia patients. J Cosmet Dermatol 2018. https://doi.org/10.1111/jocd.12810.

46. Gkini M-A, Kouskoukis A-E, Tripsianis G, et al. Study of platelet-rich plasma injections in the treatment of androgenetic alopecia through an one-year period. J Cutan Aesthet Surg 2014;7(4):213–9.

47. Ince B, Yildirim MEC, Dadaci M, et al. Comparison of the Efficacy of Homologous and Autologous Platelet-Rich Plasma (PRP) for Treating Androgenic Alopecia. Aesthet Plast Surg 2018;42(1):297–303.

48. James R, Chetry R, Subramanian V, et al. Efficacy of activated 3X platelet-rich plasma in the treatment of androgenic alopecia. J Stem Cells 2016;11(4):191–9.

49. Khatu SS, More YE, Gokhale NR, et al. Platelet-rich plasma in androgenic alopecia: myth or an effective tool. J Cutan Aesthet Surg 2014;7(2):107–10.

50. Marwah M, Godse K, Patil S, et al. Is there sufficient research data to use platelet-rich plasma in dermatology? Int J Trichology 2014;6(1):35–6.

51. Schiavone G, Raskovic D, Greco J, et al. Platelet-rich plasma for androgenetic alopecia: a pilot study. Dermatol Surg 2014;40(9):1010–9.

52. Singhal P, Agarwal S, Dhot PS, et al. Efficacy of platelet-rich plasma in treatment of androgenic alopecia. Asian J Transfus Sci 2015;9(2):159–62.

53. Starace M, Alessandrini A, D'Acunto C, et al. Platelet-rich plasma on female androgenetic alopecia: Tested on 10 patients. J Cosmet Dermatol 2019;18(1):59–64.

54. Qu Q, Shi P, Yi Y, et al. Efficacy of Platelet-rich Plasma for Treating Androgenic Alopecia of Varying Grades. Clin Drug Investig 2019;39(9):865–72.

55. Kachhawa D, Vats G, Sonare D, et al. A spilt head study of efficacy of placebo versus platelet-rich plasma injections in the treatment of androgenic alopecia. J Cutan Aesthet Surg 2017;10(2):86–9.

56. Bruce AJ, Pincelli TP, Heckman MG, et al. A Randomized, Controlled Pilot Trial Comparing Platelet-Rich Plasma to Topical Minoxidil Foam for Treatment of Androgenic Alopecia in Women. Dermatol Surg 2020;46(6):826–32.

57. Pakhomova EE. Morphological Substantiation of Clinical Efficacy of Platelet Rich Plasma in the Treatment of Androgenetic Alopecia. Int J Biomed 2018;8(4):317–20.

58. Shetty VH, Goel S. Dermoscopic pre- and post-treatment evaluation in patients with androgenetic alopecia on platelet-rich plasma-A prospective study. J Cosmet Dermatol 2018. https://doi.org/10.1111/jocd.12845.

59. Gupta AK, Bamimore MA, Foley KA. Efficacy of non-surgical treatments for androgenetic alopecia in men and women: a systematic review with network meta-analyses, and an assessment of evidence quality. J Dermatol Treat 2020;1–11. https://doi.org/10.1080/09546634.2020.1749547.

60. Ahmad M. Comparison of tissue loss by different punches: A new A-design. J Cosmet Dermatol 2019;18(1):303–7.

61. Ayatollahi A, Hosseini H, Shahdi M, et al. Platelet-rich plasma by single spin process in male pattern androgenetic alopecia: is it an effective treatment? Indian Dermatol Online J 2017;8(6):460–4.

62. Ku M-C, Teh L-S, Chen P-M, et al. Synergistic effect of platelet-rich plasma injections and scalp lifting in androgenetic alopecia. Clin Dermatol 2018;36(5):673–9.

63. Jha AK, Udayan UK, Roy PK, et al. Original article: Platelet-rich plasma with microneedling in androgenetic alopecia along with dermoscopic pre- and post-treatment evaluation. J Cosmet Dermatol 2018;17(3):313–8.

64. Takikawa M, Nakamura S, Nakamura S, et al. Enhanced effect of platelet-rich plasma containing a new carrier on hair growth. Dermatol Surg 2011;37(12):1721–9.

65. Kang J-S, Zheng Z, Choi MJ, et al. The effect of CD34+ cell-containing autologous platelet-rich plasma injection on pattern hair loss: a preliminary study. J Eur Acad Dermatol Venereol 2014;28(1):72–9.

66. Arora R, Shukla S. Injectable-platelet-rich fibrin-smart blood with stem cells for the treatment of alopecia: a report of three patients. Int J Trichology 2019;11(3):128–31.

67. Shashank B, Bhushan M. Injectable Platelet-Rich Fibrin (PRF): The newest biomaterial and its use in various dermatological conditions in our practice: A case series. J Cosmet Dermatol 2020. https://doi.org/10.1111/jocd.13742.

68. Schiavone G, Paradisi A, Ricci F, et al. Injectable Platelet-, Leukocyte-, and Fibrin-Rich Plasma (iL-PRF) in the Management of Androgenetic Alopecia. Dermatol Surg 2018;44(9):1183–90.

69. Sasse K, Ackerman E, Brandt J. Complex wounds treated with MatriStem xenograft material: case series and cost analysis.OA Surgery. OA Surg 2013;1(1):3.

70. Pakhomova EE, Smirnova IO. Comparative evaluation of the clinical efficacy of prp-therapy, minoxidil, and their combination with immunohistochemical study of the dynamics of cell proliferation in the treatment of men with androgenetic alopecia. Int J Mol Sci 2020;21(18). https://doi.org/10.3390/ijms21186516.

71. Alves R, Grimalt R. Platelet-rich plasma in combination with 5% minoxidil topical solution and 1 mg oral finasteride for the treatment of androgenetic alopecia: a randomized placebo-controlled, double-blind, half-head study. Dermatol Surg 2018;44(1):126–30.

72. Stevens HP, Donners S, de Bruijn J. Introducing platelet-rich stroma: platelet-rich plasma (PRP) and stromal vascular fraction (SVF) combined for the treatment of androgenetic alopecia. Aesthet Surg J 2018;38(8):811–22.

73. Kuka Epstein G. Isolation of adipose-derived stem cells: a primer. Hair Transplant Forum Int 2020;30(5):194–5.

74. Tosti A, Bellavista S, Iorizzo M. Alopecia areata: A long term follow-up study of 191 patients. J Am Acad Dermatol 2006;55(3):438–41.

75. Almohanna HM, Ahmed AA, Griggs JW, et al. Platelet-rich plasma in the treatment of alopecia areata: a review. J Investig Dermatol Symp Proc 2020;20(1):S45–9.

76. El Taieb MA, Ibrahim H, Nada EA, et al. Platelets rich plasma versus minoxidil 5% in treatment of alopecia areata: A trichoscopic evaluation. Dermatol Ther 2017;30(1). https://doi.org/10.1111/dth.12437.

77. Trink A, Sorbellini E, Bezzola P, et al. A randomized, double-blind, placebo- and active-controlled, half-head study to evaluate the effects of platelet-rich plasma on alopecia areata. Br J Dermatol 2013;169(3):690–4.

78. Shumez H, Prasad P, Kaviarasan P, et al. Intralesional platelet rich plasma vs intralesional triamcinolone in the treatment of alopecia areata: a comparative study. Int J Med Res Health Sci 2015;4(1):118.

79. Singh S. Role of platelet-rich plasma in chronic alopecia areata: Our centre experience. Indian J Plast Surg 2015;48(1):57–9.

80. Mubki T. Platelet-rich plasma combined with intralesional triamcinolone acetonide for the treatment of alopecia areata: A case report | Elsevier Enhanced Reader. J Dermatol Dermatol Surg 2016;20:87–90.

81. Donovan J. Successful treatment of corticosteroid-resistant ophiasis-type alopecia areata (AA) with platelet-rich plasma (PRP). JAAD Case Rep 2015;1(5):305–7.

82. d'Ovidio R. Limited Effectiveness of Platelet-Rich-Plasma Treatment on Chronic Severe Alopecia Areata. Hair Ther Transplant 2014;04(01). https://doi.org/10.4172/2167-0951.1000116.

83. Bolanča Ž, Goren A, Getaldić-Švarc B, et al. Platelet-rich plasma as a novel treatment for lichen planopillaris. Dermatol Ther 2016;29(4):233–5.

84. Jha AK. Platelet-rich plasma as an adjunctive treatment in lichen planopilaris. J Am Acad Dermatol 2019;80(5):e109–10.

85. Xu P, Wu Y, Zhou L, et al. Platelet-rich plasma accelerates skin wound healing by promoting re-epithelialization. Burns Trauma 2020. https://doi.org/10.1093/burnst/tkaa028.

86. Sakata R, Reddi AH. Platelet-rich plasma modulates actions on articular cartilage lubrication and regeneration. Tissue Eng B Rev 2016;22(5):408–19.

87. Zhao J, Harada N, Okajima K. Dihydrotestosterone inhibits hair growth in mice by inhibiting insulin-like growth factor-I production in dermal papillae. Growth Horm IGF Res 2011;21(5):260–7.

88. Kang J-I, Kim S-C, Kim M-K, et al. Effects of dihydrotestosterone on rat dermal papilla cells in vitro. Eur J Pharmacol 2015;757:74–83.

89. Kim DH, Je YJ, Kim CD, et al. Can Platelet-rich Plasma Be Used for Skin Rejuvenation? Evaluation of Effects of Platelet-rich Plasma on Human Dermal Fibroblast. Ann Dermatol 2011;23(4):424–31.

90. Uebel CO, da Silva JB, Cantarelli D, et al. The role of platelet plasma growth factors in male pattern baldness surgery. Plast Reconstr Surg 2006;118(6):1458–66 [discussion: 1467].

91. Vogt PM, Lehnhardt M, Wagner D, et al. Determination of endogenous growth factors in human wound fluid: temporal presence and profiles of secretion. Plast Reconstr Surg 1998;102(1):117–23.

92. Siah TW, Guo H, Chu T, et al. Growth factor concentrations in platelet-rich plasma for androgenetic alopecia: An intra-subject, randomized, blinded, placebo-controlled, pilot study. Exp Dermatol 2020;29(3):334–40.

93. Hom DB, Maisel RH. Angiogenic growth factors: their effects and potential in soft tissue wound healing. Ann Otol Rhinol Laryngol 1992;101(4):349–54.

94. Li W, Enomoto M, Ukegawa M, et al. Subcutaneous injections of platelet-rich plasma into skin flaps modulate proangiogenic gene expression and improve survival rates. Plast Reconstr Surg 2012;129(4):858–66.

95. Goldman BE, Fisher DM, Ringler SL. Transcutaneous PO2 of the scalp in male pattern baldness: a new piece to the puzzle. Plast Reconstr Surg 1996;97(6):1109–16 [discussion: 1117].

96. Adly MA, Assaf HA, Hussein MR, et al. Analysis of the expression pattern of glial cell line-derived neurotrophic factor, neurturin, their cognate receptors GFRalpha-1 and GFRalpha-2, and a common signal transduction element c-Ret in the human scalp skin. J Cutan Pathol 2006;33(12):799–808.

97. Li M, Liu JY, Wang S, et al. Multipotent neural crest stem cell-like cells from rat vibrissa dermal papilla induce neuronal differentiation of PC12 cells. Biomed Res Int 2014;2014:186239.

98. Botchkareva NV, Botchkarev VA, Welker P, et al. New roles for glial cell line-derived neurotrophic factor and neurturin: involvement in hair cycle control. Am J Pathol 2000;156(3):1041–53.

99. Adly MA, Assaf HA, Pertile P, et al. Expression patterns of the glial cell line-derived neurotrophic factor, neurturin, their cognate receptors GFRalpha-1, GFRalpha-2, and a common signal transduction element c-Ret in the human skin hair follicles. J Am Acad Dermatol 2008;58(2):238–50.

100. Yano K, Brown LF, Detmar M. Control of hair growth and follicle size by VEGF-mediated angiogenesis. J Clin Invest 2001;107(4):409–17.

101. Ozeki M, Tabata Y. Promoted growth of murine hair follicles through controlled release of vascular endothelial growth factor. Biomaterials 2002;23(11):2367–73.

102. Merrill MJ, Oldfield EH. A reassessment of vascular endothelial growth factor in central nervous system pathology. J Neurosurg 2005;103(5):853–68.

103. Kalaria RN, Cohen DL, Premkumar DR, et al. Vascular endothelial growth factor in Alzheimer's disease and experimental cerebral ischemia. Brain Res Mol Brain Res 1998;62(1):101–5.

104. Issa R, Krupinski J, Bujny T, et al. Vascular endothelial growth factor and its receptor, KDR, in human brain tissue after ischemic stroke. Lab Investig J Tech Methods Pathol 1999;79(4):417–25.

105. Baldo BA. Side Effects of Cytokines Approved for Therapy. Drug Saf 2014;37(11):921–43.

106. Marx RE. Platelet-rich plasma: evidence to support its use. J Oral Maxillofac Surg 2004;62(4):489–96.

107. Thomson JA, Itskovitz-Eldor J, Shapiro SS, et al. Embryonic stem cell lines derived from human blastocysts. Science 1998;282(5391):1145–7.

108. Dicke KA, van Bekkum DW. Transplantation of haemopoietic stem cell (HSC) concentrates for treatment of immune deficiency disease. Adv Exp Med Biol 1973;29(0):337–42.

109. Zuk PA, Zhu M, Ashjian P, et al. Human Adipose Tissue Is a Source of Multipotent Stem Cells. Mol Biol Cell 2002;13(12):4279–95.

110. Zuk PA. The Adipose-derived Stem Cell: Looking Back and Looking Ahead. Mol Biol Cell 2010; 21(11):1783–7.

111. Tak YJ, Lee SY, Cho AR, et al. A randomized, double-blind, vehicle-controlled clinical study of hair regeneration using adipose-derived stem cell constituent extract in androgenetic alopecia. Stem Cells Transl Med 2020;9(8):839–49.

112. Baraniak PR, McDevitt TC. Stem cell paracrine actions and tissue regeneration. Regen Med 2010; 5(1):121–43.

113. Gupta AK, Renaud HJ, Halaas Y, et al. Exosomes: A new effective non-surgical therapy for androgenetic alopecia? SKINmed 2020; 18(2):96–100.

114. Sasaki GH. Review of Human Hair Follicle Biology: Dynamics of Niches and Stem Cell Regulation for Possible Therapeutic Hair Stimulation for Plastic Surgeons. Aesthet Plast Surg 2019;43(1):253–66.

115. Zhang Y, Tomann P, Andl T, et al. Reciprocal requirements for EDA/EDAR/NF-kappaB and Wnt/ beta-catenin signaling pathways in hair follicle induction. Dev Cell 2009;17(1):49–61.

116. Zhang J, He XC, Tong W-G, et al. Bone morphogenetic protein signaling inhibits hair follicle anagen induction by restricting epithelial stem/progenitor cell activation and expansion. Stem Cells Dayt Ohio 2006;24(12):2826–39.

117. Kobielak K, Stokes N, de la Cruz J, et al. Loss of a quiescent niche but not follicle stem cells in the absence of bone morphogenetic protein signaling. Proc Natl Acad Sci U S A 2007; 104(24):10063–8.

118. Rompolas P, Greco V. Stem cell dynamics in the hair follicle niche. Semin Cell Dev Biol 2014;0:34–42.

119. Plikus MV, Mayer JA, de la Cruz D, et al. Cyclic dermal BMP signalling regulates stem cell activation during hair regeneration. Nature 2008; 451(7176):340–4.

120. Oshimori N, Fuchs E. Paracrine TGF-β signaling counterbalances BMP-mediated repression in hair follicle stem cell activation. Cell Stem Cell 2012; 10(1):63–75.

121. Plikus MV, Baker RE, Chen C-C, et al. Self-organizing and stochastic behaviors during the regeneration of hair stem cells. Science 2011; 332(6029):586–9.

122. Hsu Y-C, Pasolli HA, Fuchs E. Dynamics between stem cells, niche, and progeny in the hair follicle. Cell 2011;144(1):92–105.

123. Myung PS, Takeo M, Ito M, et al. Epithelial Wnt ligand secretion is required for adult hair follicle growth and regeneration. J Invest Dermatol 2013; 133(1):31–41.

124. Lowry WE, Blanpain C, Nowak JA, et al. Defining the impact of beta-catenin/Tcf transactivation on epithelial stem cells. Genes Dev 2005;19(13): 1596–611.

125. Leirós GJ, Attorresi AI, Balañá ME. Hair follicle stem cell differentiation is inhibited through crosstalk between Wnt/β-catenin and androgen signalling in dermal papilla cells from patients with androgenetic alopecia. Br J Dermatol 2012; 166(5):1035–42.

126. Rehman J, Traktuev D, Li J, et al. Secretion of angiogenic and antiapoptotic factors by human adipose stromal cells. Circulation 2004;109(10): 1292–8.

127. Kilroy GE, Foster SJ, Wu X, et al. Cytokine profile of human adipose-derived stem cells: expression of angiogenic, hematopoietic, and pro-inflammatory factors. J Cell Physiol 2007;212(3):702–9.

128. Kim W-S, Park B-S, Sung J-H, et al. Wound healing effect of adipose-derived stem cells: a critical role of secretory factors on human dermal fibroblasts. J Dermatol Sci 2007;48(1):15–24.

129. Shin H, Ryu HH, Kwon O, et al. Clinical use of conditioned media of adipose tissue-derived stem cells in female pattern hair loss: a retrospective case series study. Int J Dermatol 2015;54(6): 730–5.

130. Fukuoka H, Suga H. Hair Regeneration Treatment Using Adipose-Derived Stem Cell Conditioned Medium: Follow-up With Trichograms. Eplasty 2015; 15:e10.

131. Fukuoka H, Narita K, Suga H. Hair Regeneration Therapy: Application of Adipose-Derived Stem Cells. Curr Stem Cell Res Ther 2017;12(7): 531–4.

132. Narita K, Fukuoka H, Sekiyama T, et al. Sequential scalp assessment in hair regeneration therapy using an adipose-derived stem cell-conditioned medium. Dermatol Surg 2020; 46(6):819–25.

133. Gimble Jeffrey M, Katz Adam J, Bunnell Bruce A. Adipose-derived stem cells for regenerative medicine. Circ Res 2007;100(9):1249–60.

134. Perez-Meza D, Ziering C, Sforza M, et al. Hair follicle growth by stromal vascular fraction-enhanced adipose transplantation in baldness. Stem Cells Cloning Adv Appl 2017;10:1–10.

135. Kuka G, Epstein J, Aronowitz J, et al. Cell Enriched Autologous Fat Grafts to Follicular Niche Improves Hair Regrowth in Early Androgenetic Alopecia. Aesthet Surg J 2020;40(6):NP328–39.

136. Gentile P, Scioli MG, Bielli A, et al. Stem cells from human hair follicles: first mechanical

isolation for immediate autologous clinical use in androgenetic alopecia and hair loss. Stem Cell Investig 2017;4:58.

137. Zhou L, Wang H, Jing J, et al. Regulation of hair follicle development by exosomes derived from dermal papilla cells. Biochem Biophys Res Commun 2018;500(2):325–32.

138. Cooley JE. Bone Marrow Derived MSC Exosomes for AA: The First 100 Patients. Presentation presented at the: International Society of Hair Restoration Surgeons World Congress; Oct 17-25, 2020; Virtual.

139. Zari S. The Use of Exosomes in the Management of Androgenetic Alopecia/Female Pattern Hair Loss. Presentation presented at the: International Society of Hair Restoration Surgeons World Congress; Oct 17-25, 2020; Virtual.

140. FDA. Public safety notification on exosome products. U.S. Food & Drug Administration; 2019. Available at: https://www.fda.gov/vaccinesblood-biologics/safety-availability-biologics/public-safety-notification- exosome-products.

141. Anderi R, Makdissy N, Azar A, et al. Cellular therapy with human autologous adipose-derived adult cells of stromal vascular fraction for alopecia areata. Stem Cell Res Ther 2018;9(1):141.

142. Li Y, Yan B, Wang H, et al. Hair regrowth in alopecia areata patients following Stem Cell Educator therapy. BMC Med 2015;13:87.

143. Elmaadawi IH, Mohamed BM, Ibrahim ZAS, et al. Stem cell therapy as a novel therapeutic intervention for resistant cases of alopecia areata and androgenetic alopecia. J Dermatol Treat 2018;29(5):431–40.

Energy-based Devices for Hair Loss

James T. Pathoulas, BA[a], Gretchen Bellefeuille, BS[a], Ora Raymond, BA[a],
Bisma Khalid, MBBS, FCPS[b], Ronda S. Farah, MD[a],*

KEYWORDS

- Devices • Alopecia • Photobiomodulation • Low-Level Laser Light • Fractionated Lasers
- Microneedling • Laser-Assisted Drug Deliver

KEY POINTS

- Energy based devices including fractionated lasers, photobiomodulation, and microneedling are emerging therapies for alopecia.
- Photobiomodulation (PBM), or low-level laser light, has been well studied as a treatment of androgenetic alopecia and several devices have received FDA clearance. There is sufficient evidence to recommend PBM as a treatment for androgenetic alopecia (AGA) but the devices are not typically covered by insurance.
- Microneedling is thought to promote hair growth through microscopic wounding of the skin. There is limited evidence to suggest microneedling as a first-line therapy for AGA. However, it is generally safe and early efficacy data is promising.
- Treatment with non-ablative fractionated lasers have resulted in improved hair density among those with AGA in a limited number of randomized trials. Ablative fractionated lasers have been investigated in inflammatory hair disorders with mixed results in the few published case series. Further studies are needed to determine the safety and efficacy of fractionated lasers in the treatment of AGA.
- Device-assisted drug delivery creates microscopic wounds in the epidermis, facilitating the delivery of large and hydrophilic drugs to the hair follicle. Early studies examining fractionated lasers and microneedling assisted drug delivery for AGA are promising.

INTRODUCTION

Treatment options for hair loss have traditionally been limited to topical and systemic therapies. Systemic therapies for inflammatory hair disorders are often immunosuppressive, and systemic treatment of androgenetic hair loss can cause undesired effects on sexual and reproductive health. Topical agents have a favorable side effect profile compared with systemic therapies, but many topicals have poor transcutaneous absorption, limiting their concentration and action at follicular targets in the dermis.

Limitations to traditional therapies have spurred significant interest in energy-based devices for the treatment of hair and scalp disorders, as shown by a limited but growing body of promising literature and a rapidly growing number of US Food and Drug Administration (FDA)–approved devices entering the marketplace. Energy-based devices stand apart from traditional hair loss therapies in their proposed mechanism of action and many studies show positive results with device monotherapy. Some preliminary studies have also reported an additive effect on hair growth when combining novel

[a] Department of Dermatology, University of Minnesota, 516 Delaware Street Southeast Mail Code 98, Phillips-Wangensteen Building, Suite 4- 420, Minneapolis, MN 55455, USA; [b] University of Minnesota, 420 Delaware St SE, Minneapolis, MN 55455, USA
* Corresponding author. 516 Delaware Street Southeast Mail Code 98, Phillips-Wangensteen Building, Suite 4-420, Minneapolis, MN 55455.
E-mail address: rfarah@umn.edu

Dermatol Clin 39 (2021) 447–461
https://doi.org/10.1016/j.det.2021.04.002

energy-based device treatment and traditional topical therapy.

This article covers the use of photobiomodulation (PBM), microneedling, laser therapy (including laser-assisted drug delivery [LADD]), and radiofrequency (RF) in the treatment of hair loss.

PHOTOBIOMODULATION
Background

PBM, or low-level laser therapy (LLLT), was discovered at the Semmelweis Medical University in Hungary more than 50 years ago by Endre Mester, who aimed to destroy tumors in rats with a ruby laser.[1,2] Although the laser was ineffective against tumors, hair growth was noted on the treated areas. Since that time, the use of other light modalities including PBM in the management of hair loss has expanded. PBM or photobiomodulation therapy are now recognized as the desired terms for this light application.[3]

Although the mechanism of PBM is not fully understood, it has been theorized that PBM may have an effect on cell-signaling pathways, transcriptional processes, and modification of gene expression.[4] Red (600-700 nm) and near infrared (760-1000+ nm) light is thought to cause increased ATP production via photon-mediated disinhibition of cytochrome c oxidase in the mitochondrial respiratory chain (**Figure 1**).[4,5] In addition, the light from these devices increases nitric oxide bioavailability, stimulating keratinocyte

growth (**Figure 1**).[6] These various intracellular events trigger cell division and differentiation, which initiates the transition of follicular stem cells to progenitor cells, and then hair matrix cells. Once cells have developed into matrix cells, the hair follicle enters anagen (growth) phase, which leads to increased overall scalp hair; this proposed mechanism has primarily been studied in androgenetic alopecia (AGA) as a primary disease model (**Figure 2**).[4] For autoimmune diseases such as alopecia areata (AA), where macrophage activation is involved in pathogenesis, there is considerable evidence that PBM can inhibit the release of proinflammatory cytokines.[4] PBM also inhibits apoptosis of cells through the upregulation of anti-apoptotic proteins, which can be used in the treatment of chemotherapy-induced alopecia.[7]

Photobiomodulation Devices

PBM was first FDA approved in 2007 for the treatment of AGA.[8] For hair loss treatment, coherent and noncoherent light sources have been used in the development of commercially available hair loss devices.[9] Typically, the noncoherent light sources used include light-emitting diodes (LEDs) and the coherent light sources are laser diodes.[9] The Revian Red (Durham, NC), uses 100% LEDs with two different wavelengths (620 nm and 660 nm) of light to promote an optimal environment for hair growth.[10] Devices have also used a combination of LEDs and laser diodes; for example, the iGrow

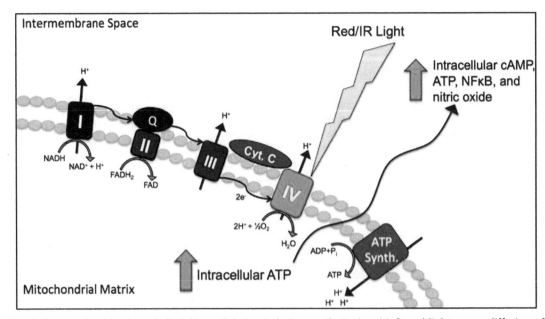

Fig. 1. Proposed mechanism of photobiomodulation in hair growth. Red and infrared light causes diffusion of hydrogen across the inner mitochondrial membrane, facilitating production of ATP and increasing intracellular transcription factors including NFkB. (*Courtesy* of MacKenzie Griffith).

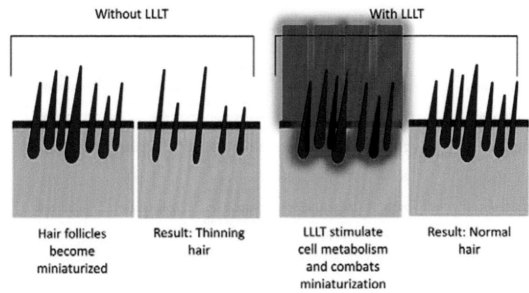

Without LLLT

With LLLT

Hair follicles become miniaturized

Result: Thinning hair

LLLT stimulate cell metabolism and combats miniaturization

Result: Normal hair

Fig. 2. Depiction of proposed mechanism of photobiomodulation in androgenetic alopecia, also known as LLLT (low-level light therapy). *Courtesy* of Revian Red (Durham, NC).

Hair Growth System (Boca Raton, FL), the iRestore Essential (Irvine, CA), and the iRestore Professional (Irvine, CA). With regard to lasers, most devices have been marketed at 655 nm +/− 5, the first of which was the HairMax LaserComb (Lexington International, Boca Raton, FL).[11] Of note, there are 2 devices on the market, Theradome ProLH80 and Theradome Evo LH40, that emit light at 678 nm light.[11] Within each laser source, each diode has the power capacity of 5 mW.[11] The number of laser diodes within a device varies from 9 to 304, creating total outputs from 45 mW all the way up to 1520 mW. The duration of treatment and frequency also vary among these devices. Treatment times can range from as little as 90 seconds three days a week to 30 minutes every other day (**Table 1**). However, the optimal energy and treatment time for hair growth enhancement is unknown.

Many of these devices are available directly to the consumer, within salons, spas, and medical offices, and few are obtained through authorized medical professionals. Device design includes combs, helmets, caps, bands, in-office units, and at-home units (see **Figure 3** and **Table 1**). Some devices include hair-parting teeth, present in the HairMax LaserBand and LaserComb, that allow light to reach the scalp and follicles directly.[12] Devices may include features such as automatic treatment times, sounds or vibrations to alert users when to move the device, and safety controls (see **Table 1**). Revian Red utilizes a phone app that can connect wirelessly to the cap. This app allows the users to start and stop their sessions each day, set up reminders, compare photographs, and track

their hair growth progress. These products have a wide range of costs, some around $199.00 and others around $3000.00.

Clinical Evidence for Management of Hair Loss

Androgenetic alopecia

The first randomized, sham-device–controlled study was performed with the HairMax LaserComb® in the treatment of AGA.[8] The study included 123 men ranging from ages 30 to 60 years who had a diagnosis of AGA for at least 12 months. The participants were instructed to use the comb three times a week for 6 months and were assessed at the end of the study duration for evidence of new hair growth and analysis of hair clippings and hair counts. Those treated with the HairMax LaserComb® had on average a +19.8 hairs/cm^2 increase in terminal hair density. Subjects using the sham device had an average decrease of −7.6 hairs/cm^2. The light treated hair group had a statistically significant increase in hair density when compared to the sham group.[8]

A subsequent study evaluating the use of the HairMax LaserComb® was performed in 128 men and 141 women.[13] Participants were randomized into either a treatment (laser) group or placebo (sham) group. The study occurred over the duration of 26 weeks with an end goal of evaluating changes in terminal hair density from the baseline and 26-week follow-up. At assessment, participants in the laser group showed a significant improvement in hair density compared with the sham group. Hair counts improved from baseline

Table 1
Select of US Food and Drug Administration–approved photobiomodulation devices

Device	FDA Cleared	Light Source	Design	Treatment	Approximate Cost ($)
CapillusUltra	2015	82 laser diodes	Hands-free sports cap	6 min daily	999.00
CapillusPlus	2016	202 laser diodes	Hands-free sports cap	6 min daily	1799.00
CapillusPro	2016	272 laser diodes	Hands-free sports cap	6 min daily	2999.00
CapillusUltra+	2019	112 laser diodes	Hands-free sports cap	6 min daily	1199.00
Capillus X+	2019	244 laser diodes	Hands-free sports cap	6 min daily	2899.00
HairMax Laser 272 PowerFlex Cap	2018	272 laser diodes	Hands-free sports cap	15 min, 3 times a week	1899.00
HairMax LaserBand 82	2014	82 laser diodes	Headband	Minimum 90 s, 3 times a week	799.00
HairMax LaserBand 41	2014	41 laser diodes	Headband	Minimum 3 min, 3 times a week	549.00
HairMax Ultima 12 LaserComb	2011	12 laser diodes	Comb	8 min, 3 times a week	399.00
HairMax Ultima 9 Classic LaserComb	2011	9 laser diodes	Comb	11 min, 3 times a week	199.00
iGrow Hair Growth Laser System	2012	21 laser diodes and 30 LEDs	Hands-free helmet	25 min, every other day	449.00
iRestore Essential	2016	21 laser diodes and 30 LEDs	Hands-free helmet	25 min, every other day	695.00
iRestore Professional	2019	82 laser diodes and 200 LEDs	Hands-free helmet	25 min, every other day	1195.00
Theradome Pro LH80	2017	80 laser diodes	Hands-free helmet	20 min, 2 times a week	895.00
Theradome Evo LH40	2018	40 laser diodes	Hands-free helmet	20 min, 4 times a week	595.00
Revian Red Hair Growth System	2017	100% LED, 660 and 620 nm wavelengths	Hands-free helmet	10 min daily	995.00
LaserCap LCPRO	2015	224 laser diodes	Hands-free sports cap	15–30 min, 2 times a week	2995.00
LaserCap300 MC2	2015	304 laser diodes	Hands-free cap	Not available	Not available
NutraStim Laser Hair Comb	2015	12 laser diodes	Comb	8 min, 3 times a week	279.00
illumniflow 272 Laser Cap	2017	272 laser diodes	Hands-free cap	30 min, 3 times a week	799.00
illumniflow 148 Laser Cap	2017	148 laser diodes	Hands-free cap	30 min, 3 times a week	549.00
Kiierr 148 Pro Laser Cap	2018	148 laser diodes	Hands-free sports cap	30 min, every other day	595.00
Kiierr 272 Premier Laser Cap	2018	272 laser diodes	Hands-free sports cap	30 min, every other day	845.00

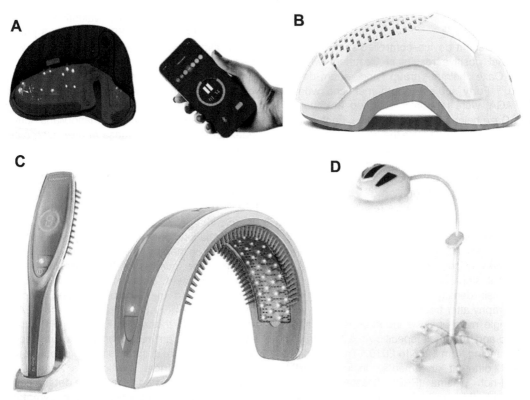

Fig. 3. Examples of in-home and in-office devices In-Home Revian Red. Courtesy of Revian Red (Durham, NC) Theradome. Courtesy of Theradome (Silicon Valley, CA) HairMax. Courtesy of HairMax (Lexington International, Boca Raton, FL) In-Office Capillus. Courtesy of Curallux, LLC (Miami, FL).

by approximately 20 to 25 hairs/cm². Both studies analyzing the HairMax LaserComb® demonstrated that PBM may be a promising therapy for men and women with AGA.[13] Similar results were reported in a study of 28 male and 7 female participants who were instructed to use the LaserMax Hair-Comb® every other day for five to ten minutes at a time.[14] Temporary shedding similar to the initial shed that patients experience when using minoxidil was reported. This shedding subsided after two months and overall improvement of hair counts and hair tensile strength was observed after six months of treatment.[13]

The iGrow hands-free helmet device (Boca Raton, FL) was FDA cleared in 2012. This device incorporates both LEDs and lasers. The device was studied in 44 male participants with AGA, who were recruited and randomly assigned to either the treatment or sham-device group.[15] The duration of the study was 16 weeks; each subject used the at-home device for 25 minutes every other day. At the end of the treatment duration, researchers examined baseline and posttreatment photographs, looking for any improvement in overall hair counts. Among participants who were assigned to the treatment group, there was a significant

increase in terminal hair counts and the hairs appeared to be darker and thicker. The average percentage increase in the terminal hairs of participants in the treatment group was 35% compared with the placebo group. The device produced similar results in an identical study of women with AGA.[16]

The Capillus272 Pro (Miami, FL) laser helmet was first evaluated in 44 female participants with AGA.[17] This 17-week study consisted of 2 groups: a laser (active) group and a placebo (sham) group. The The intervention group self-treated group self-treated with a 650-nm dome device for 30 minutes every other day. Participants in the sham group were also instructed to self-treat for 30 minutes every other day. At the end of the 17-week study duration, hair counts were compared with baseline by examining photographs. When comparing the 2 groups, the results were statistically significant, with a 51% increase in hair counts in the treatment group versus the placebo group.[17]

A clinical trial examining the Revian Red (Durham, NC) LED device in 18 male and female participants with AGA over 16 weeks reported growth of 26.3 more hairs per square centimeter on average in the treatment arm compared with the placebo (sham) group. Participants in the placebo group continued to observe hair loss over the study period.[18]

A single sham-device–controlled study reported additional positive results in treatment with an PBM Oaze helmet group and sham-device group.[19] Forty subjects, both men and women with AGA, were randomly assigned to either an LLLT Oaze helmet or a sham device. Each participant was instructed to use the device daily, 18 minutes each time, for 24 weeks. Results showed that patients who used the PBM helmet had greater increase in hair thickness, though subject self-assessments did not align.[19]

A study reporting negative results investigated the efficacy of PBM in seven patients, one man and six women.[20] Over a study duration of 3 to 6 months, participants were treated with PBM for 20 minutes twice a week. Overall, there was no significant improvement as measured by hair count, hair density, and assessment of global photography after treatment.[19]

A single meta-analysis incorporated 30 male-specific and 10 female-specific AGA studies with dates ranging from 1986 to 2019.[7] They identified several different treatments, including PBM, platelet-rich plasma (PRP), finasteride 1 mg, dutasteride 0.5 mg, topical minoxidil 2%, topical minoxidil 5%, and topical bimatoprost. After analysis, each of these treatments resulted in improvement in average hair counts compared with placebo groups; however, PBM and PRP were significantly more effective.[6]

A comprehensive literature review examined the safety and effectiveness of PBM in both men and women with AGA.[21] The analysis included 10 randomized and controlled studies, most of which compared PBM monotherapy treatment with a sham (placebo) device. One of the studies used topical minoxidil 5% solution as the treatment group and the other study compared PBM with no treatment. Five different types of laser devices were used among the studies and treatment durations ranged from 16 to 26 weeks. In addition, frequency of treatment and laser parameters varied. Assessment was based on either the Hamilton-Norwood scale or the Ludwig-Savin scale. In all of the studies, participants who were treated with PBM devices achieved increases in hair growth, terminal hair counts, and overall scalp hair coverage with only minimal adverse events noted in a few studies.

Cicatricial alopecias

Two studies directly assessed the effectiveness of PBM for the treatment of cicatricial or scarring alopecia, including frontal fibrosing alopecia (FFA) and lichen planopilaris (LPP). The first study was a 6-month prospective study evaluating the effectiveness of Ledmedical LED devices in 8 participants diagnosed with LPP.[22] The devices were used at high power for 15 minutes every day for a total of 6 months. All patients showed improvement after treatment, with an overall reduction of symptoms, perifollicular hyperkeratosis, erythema, and an average Lichen Planopilaris Activity Index (LPPAI) score decrease of 0.87. Compared with baseline assessment, there was an increase in the thickness of terminal hair at both 3 and 6 months.[22] A second study assessed the efficacy of PBM as a treatment for patients with LPP/FFA.[23] The study included 16 women, 8 with LPP and 8 with FFA. All participants were treated with LED irradiations once a week for 10 weeks. After 10 weeks of therapy, there was a significant increase in the number of thick hairs within the area of treatment. Standardized scoring assessments included the Frontal Fibrosing Alopecia Severity Score (FFASS) and LPPAI score. After treatment, both those with FFA and LPP experienced a significant reduction in their respective scores.[23] Due to a small sample population in both studies, more participants should be assessed in future studies for a true determination of efficacy. Similar reduction in scalp symptoms and improvement in hair growth have been reported in case report format.[24]

Side Effects

Few adverse events have been reported in studies evaluating the effect of PBM on hair growth. The most common side effects include hair shedding, xerosis, erythema, pruritus, irritation, scalp tenderness, warm sensation, urticaria, and acne. As with any light-based device, patients should be advised to avoid directly aiming the laser light into their eyes. Continued surveillance of these devices and long-term patient health is important.

Limitations and Future Directions

Overall, the literature is supportive of the use of PBM for the mangement of AGA. The remaining uses are off-label and further studies are needed. Despite significant clinical research and FDA approval, the most effective parameters and device design for hair growth remain unclear. The need to identify the most efficacious wavelength, power, treatment time, treatment frequency, and light source remains. In addition, PBM devices are not usually covered by insurance, thereby limiting access to patients with ability to purchase out of pocket. A greater understanding of the optimal settings between hair and skin types is lacking. Although PBM for AGA has been the most widely studied, the role of PBM in cicatricial alopecias is promising.

MICRONEEDLING
Overview

Microneedling has been a trending treatment option for the management of alopecia. Traditionally, microneedling microneedling is used off-label for hair loss has been utilized as either monotherapy or as a method of drug delivery. The precise mechanism of microneedling in the role of hair growth is unknown but is thought to involve microtraumas that stimulate the Wnt/β-catenin pathway, which promotes hair growth.[25] When used as a method of drug delivery, microneedling creates microscopic punctures, allowing transfollicular and transepidermal delivery of topical agents.[26]

Types of Microneedling Devices

There are two major classes of microneedling devices: rollers and powered devices. The Dermaroller®, which is a nonelectrical hand-held device with 192 needles that range from 0.5 to 1.5 mm in length.[27] Dermarollers possess a rotating headpiece with multiple needles that, when rolled on skin, penetrate the stratum corneum and generate microconduits (holes) that cause minimal epidermal trauma.[28] In contrast, powered devices such as the Dermapen typically have 9 to 12 needles and function as an electrically powered device that delivers spring-loaded punches in a stamping motion.[29]

Microneedling Monotherapy Treatments

Microneedling monotherapy has shown promise though very preliminary results for hair regeneration. A murine model microneedling study examining the optimal depth of microneedle penetration and number of total treatments reported hair growth and significant upregulation of hair growth transcription factors, including Wnt3a, β-catenin, vascular endothelial growth factor, and Wnt10b, at a depth of both 0.25 mm and 0.5 mm with a treatment period of 5 weeks.[30] Microneedling monotherapy trials in humans have reported similarly positive results.

A single-group open-label pilot study examined 3 dermaroller sessions over 6 months in 14 males with pattern hair loss, 29 females with pattern hair loss, and 7 females with TE.[31] Patients continued concomitant hair loss treatments during the study. A 1.5 mm microneedle depth was used and pinpoint bleeding was the procedural endpoint. All participants had increased hair density and diameter by trichoscopic assessment. No serious adverse events were reported.[31] A case series examining 15 dermaroller sessions over 24 weeks in 4 males with longstanding AGA reported improvement in all participants on investigator assessment of scalp photography without significant adverse events.[32] Patients had longstanding history of treatment with oral finasteride and topical minoxidil, which they continued during and after treatment. The treatment response was sustained at 18 month follow-up.[32] Additionally, a randomized split-scalp trial examining a radiofrequency equipped microneedling device reported similarly positive results and is discussed in more detail in the radiofrequency section of this chapter.[33]

Microneedle Assisted Drug Delivery

A key limitation of topical treatments is poor transcutaneous absorption. The stratum corneum serves as a physical barrier to molecules greater than 500 Daltons and is rich in lipids and ceramides, limiting penetration of hydrophilic agents.[34] As a result, the number of efficacious topical treatments is limited by molecular properties and effective formulations need to have high concentration of active agent to drive diffusion across the skin.

Minoxidil is the only topical treatment for AGA approved by the FDA. Its inhibition of potassium channels on arteriolar smooth muscle causes a direct vasodilatory effect.[35] Minoxidil promotes follicular transition to anagen (growing) phase at the dermal papilla, but its precise mechanism of action remains unknown. Recent in vitro models show minoxidil indirectly stimulates proliferation of dermal papilla cells.[36] Future studies are needed to further elucidate the biochemical pathways involved in minoxidil mediated anagen phase promotion.

Minoxidil is hydrophilic and commercially available in foam and liquid solutions that both utilize an alcohol-based vehicle, further lowering bioavailability of topical preparations and potentially contributing to contact dermatitis.[35] A number of preliminary studies have examined microneedle enhanced delivery of minoxidil and other drugs, some of which are highlighted in this chapter.

A case series of three patients with AA were treated with a microneedling device and topical application of aerosolized triamcinolone acetonide, meso-solution (growth factors, amino acids, mineral, etc.), and minoxidil 2-5%.[37] All patients showed improvement in hair growth after six treatment sessions ranging from 50% to upwards of 90% improvement. However, the patients continued systemic therapies, making interpretation of results difficult.[37] A similar case series examined three sessions of microneedle assisted triamcinolone delivery in two patients with treatment-resistant AA over three weeks.[38] With each session, improvement was observed and after the three-month follow up no recurrence was seen.[38]

Microneedling has been described in combination with light-based treatments in a split-scalp study comparing three months of microneedling monotherapy and microneedling with photodynamic therapy (PDT) in alopecia totalis (AT).[39] The study utilized global photography and scalp biopsies. There was no significant difference in hair growth or histological findings between treatment areas. Combination PDT and microneedling is not likely superior to standalone microneedling in the treatment of AT but more studies are needed.

The use of microneedle assisted drug delivery has also been described in the treatment of AGA. A randomized control trial in 100 males with AGA evaluated compared once weekly microneedle assisted minoxidil 5% delivery with minoxidil 5% monotherapy.[40] Both groups applied minoxidil twice daily. After 12 weeks, the combination treatment group experienced significantly greater hair counts than the minoxidil monotherapy group. Patients who underwent microneedling treatment reported higher satisfaction with treatment than those using only minoxidil. No significant adverse effects were reported in either group.[40] Similar positive results were reported in an investigator blinded RCT examining electrodynamic microneedling in 60 men with AGA.[41] Subjects were randomly assigned to topical minoxidil 5%, electrodynamic microneedling, or combination treatment. Microneedling consisted of 12 sessions over 24 weeks. Those who underwent microneedle assisted delivery of minoxidil had an average 19.5cm^2 greater hair density than those using topical minoxidil and 14.9cm^2 greater hair density than those using microneedling. Adverse events among those microneedling included infection, seborrheic dermatitis, and scalp itch.[41] Smaller studies have similarly reported positive treatment effects with microneedle assisted minoxidil delivery in the treatment of AGA.[42]

Other microneedling combination treatment include incorporation of platelet-rich plasma (PRP), another increasingly popular treatment option for AGA. PRP is typically injected in the scalp after centrifugation of whole blood from the patient. Recent studies have examined microneedle assisted PRP delivery in combination with PRP injection.[43,44] However, more data and standardized techniques for comparison with standalone PRP and isolated microneedling are necessary.

Summary

Microneedling may have a role in hair loss management. However, the evidence supporting its use is preliminary. The potential to be combined with other treatment modalities including topical drugs is promising. However, future research is needed to determine optimal monotherapy treatment regimens and further identity potential topical agents that are good candidates for microneedling-assisted drug delivery.

OVERVIEW OF FRACTIONATED LASER THERAPY FOR HAIR LOSS
Introduction

Use of fractionated lasers for skin rejuvenation is well described and is considered a noninvasive alternative to cosmetic surgery. However, fractionated lasers are the most intensive energy-based devices used for hair loss. Observations of hair growth following skin injury led to the theory that injury at the level of the dermis near the base of the follicle with laser light could stimulate hair growth.[45] There is a growing body of literature that supports this theory. This article reviews the basics of fractional laser therapy and its application in hair and scalp disorders.

Fractionated lasers emit infrared and near-infrared light in a grid pattern, causing selective thermal injury that spares surrounding healthy skin, facilitating healing and minimizing recovery time. Growth factors and cytokines released in response to tissue injury stimulate hair restoration through proliferation and differentiation of progenitor cells in follicular units.[46] Laser therapy has been shown to increase the proportion of follicles in anagen phase through upregulation of the Wnt/β-catenin signaling pathway.[47] Both ablative and nonablative fractionated lasers have been investigated as treatments for hair loss.

Nonablative Laser Therapy

Fractionated 1550-nm erbium-glass and 1927-nm thulium lasers have been studied as monotherapy to both promote and induce hair growth in patients with AGA and AA.[48–51] Treatment of alopecia with laser therapy requires a balance between causing sufficient thermal injury to stimulate hair growth and preventing fibrosis that destroys hair stem cells or permanently disrupts follicular ultrastructure. Relative to ablative lasers, nonablative fractionated lasers cause less tissue damage and disruption of existing terminal hairs, and lead to fewer pigmentary changes in patients with dark skin types.[46]

Most studies evaluating the use of nonablative laser therapy to treat alopecia have used the 1550-nm fractional erbium-glass laser (**Figure 4**). A recent study of 47 patients with AGA found that 10 treatment sessions with a 1550-nm fractional erbium-glass laser spaced 2 weeks apart resulted in significantly increased hair diameter and density in all women and men with Hamilton-Norwood scores II to IV.[52] Similar results have been reported in female patients with pattern hair loss. A prospective, single-blinded trial found treatment with 1550-nm fractional erbium-glass laser led to increased hair density and diameter in 27 women with FPHL. The study investigators noted that, despite treatment of hair loss on the entire scalp, all participants had particularity robust regrowth along the frontal hairline.[48]

Use of thulium laser has been investigated as a treatment for AGA. Biopsy following treatment with a 1927-nm fractionated thulium laser on murine skin revealed a robust dermal inflammatory response without deposition of disordered collagen in perifollicular areas or other signs of follicular fibrosis.[49] In 10 men with AGA, 12 sessions of the 1927-nm fractionated thulium laser over 12 weeks resulted in increased hair density and thickness. However, the full treatment effect was not maintained at 3-month follow-up.[49]

Several case reports and smaller studies have investigated treatment of AA and alopecia universalis (AU) with nonablative laser therapy. Use of 1550-nm fractional erbium-glass laser on the scalp of 6 patients with treatment-resistant AA resulted in physician-rated improvement in global photography after 1 to 9 treatment sessions, including a dramatic improvement in a single patient with AU.[50] Patches treated with laser therapy showed stable growth without evidence of recurrence at the end of the study.[50] Smaller case series and case reports show similar success in the treatment of long-standing resistant AA with nonablative laser therapy, including 2 patients with ophiasis (**Table 2**).[51,53–55]

Ablative Laser Therapy

CO_2 lasers vaporize water in the skin, creating thousands of microscopic conical channels of thermal injury. The invention of ablative laser therapy was central to the theory of LADD, which is described separately here. More literature to support the use of ablative laser treatment of monotherapy in alopecia is needed. However, clinical improvement following monotherapy with CO_2 ablative laser therapy has been reported in individual cases of dissecting cellulitis, secondary cicatricial alopecias, and autosomal recessive woolly hair/hypotrichosis.[53] A single study examining fractional neodymium–yttrium-aluminum-garnet (Nd:YAG) and fractional ablative CO_2 lasers in 32 patients with AA did not find a significant increase in hair density or count.[56] Although pilot data examining ablative laser therapy for hair loss disorders are promising, there is a possibility of destroying the hair follicle with an ablative laser and more research is needed.

Limitations and Future Directions

Future large-scale studies examining the safety and efficacy of laser monotherapy for alopecia are needed. Support for laser therapy in the literature is needed for this to reach the appropriate level of evidence for routine care in the United States. If efficacious, then insurance coverage of these procedures, which are costly out of pocket, may be considered. Despite these limitations, preliminary studies suggest fractionated lasers may be effective for treatment-resistant alopecia.

LASER-ASSISTED DRUG DELIVERY
Introduction

Many prefer topical therapies for the treatment of hair and scalp disorders, as they have fewer side effects than systemic therapies and are easy to use. Ablation of the stratum corneum with a fractionated laser reduces the rate-limiting step of topical drug diffusion, assisting the delivery of large and hydrophilic molecules to dermal structures. The use of LADD has been successfully described with various agents, including triamcinolone acetonide, methyl aminolevulinate (MAL),

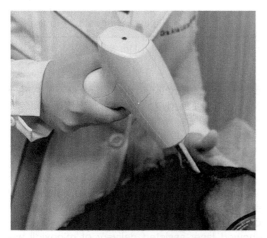

Fig. 4. RESURFX (non ablative fractional erbium laser) laser piece is passed over areas of hair thinning. *Courtesy of Dr. Ana Lucia Junqueira.*

Table 2
Studies examining fractional laser monotherapy for alopecia

Study Author	Level of Evidence	Laser	Participants and Condition	Outcome
Lee et al,[43] 2011	3	1550-nm erbium-glass	28 women with AGA	Increased terminal hair density and diameter after 5 mo of treatment
Yoo et al,[35] 2010	5		1 man with AA	Complete regrowth of hair after 24 treatments
Kim et al,[30] 2010	3		20 men with AGA	No significant change in terminal hair density and diameter, but clinical improvement
Eckert et al,[46] 2017	5		5 patients with AA	All AA patches resolved within 3 mo of treatment
Tsai et al,[72] 2016	5		1 man with AA	Split scalp, half treated with laser + ILK vs ILK. Improvement with combination only
Alhattab et al,[47] 2020	3		47 patients with AGA	10 treatment sessions, 2 wk apart, improvement in density and diameter for all women and men with HN II–IV
Mendieta-Eckert,[73] 2020	3		6 patients with AA	All patients had clinical improvement after median 3 sessions
Cho et al,[48] 2013	5	1550-nm erbium-glass and 10,600-nm CO_2	17 patients with scarring and nonscarring disorders	Improvement in AA with nonablative laser, but not ablative. AR hypotrichosis improved with both ablative and nonablative laser
Cho et al,[44] 2018	2	1927-nm thulium	10 men with AGA	12 sessions at 1-wk intervals resulted in significant increases in hair density and thickness after 5 mo of treatment
Yalici-Armagan et al,[51] 2016	3	10,600-nm CO_2 and Nd:YAG	32 patients with AA	Neither Nd:YAG nor fractional CO_2 lasers increased mean hair count or density within patches of active disease

Abbreviations: AR, autosomal recessive; HN, Hamilton-Norwood; ILK, intralesional Kenalog; Nd:YAG, neodymium–yttrium-aluminum-garnet.

and 5-fluorouracil.[57] The use of LADD to facilitate the delivery of topical agents to follicular structures in the dermis and hypodermis is of interest to augment existing therapies and develop novel treatments for hair and scalp disorders. However, there is no standard of care or protocols for LADD and treatment is primarily research based. The most frequently published medications used in LADD are briefly examined here.

Minoxidil

A few in vivo studies have examined laser assisted delivery of minoxidil in the treatment of alopecia and it remains an active area of research (**Figure. 5**).[58] The first study to examine LADD of minoxidil was conducted in murine and porcine skin models that were pre-treated with a 2940-nm erbium -yttrium -aluminum -garnet (Er -YAG) laser, resulting in a twofold increase of minoxidil concentration at the hair follicle compared to no laser therapy.[59]

An open-label interventional trial examining 6 sessions of LADD of minoxidil 5% with fractional CO_2 laser in 45 men with AGA over 12 weeks showed laser-assisted delivery of minoxidil was superior to both topical therapy and laser only with respect to thin hair count and thickness of

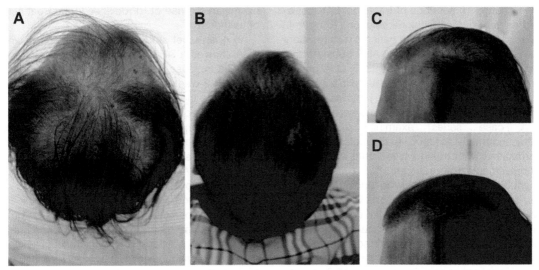

Fig. 5. Single patient with androgenetic alopecia before (2A, 2C) and after (2B, 2D) treatment with laser assisted drug delivery. *Courtesy* of Dr. Ana Lucia Junqueira.

thin hairs.[60] However, no difference in total hairs or hair diameter was observed between groups. There was no significant difference in physician-rated assessment of global scalp photography or patient self-reported satisfaction between the laser-assisted minoxidil group, laser-only group, and minoxidil-only group.

Similar results were reported in an investigator-blinded, split-scalp study evaluating the efficacy of 12 sessions of CO_2 fractionated laser-assisted minoxidil delivery over 24 weeks in 29 men with AGA compared with minoxidil alone.[61] Both hair density and diameter were greater on the treatment area that received combination laser and minoxidil therapies. Physicians rated combination-treated scalp higher on global photography evaluation, and patients' self-reported satisfaction with hair growth was significantly greater on combination-treated scalp. No serious adverse effects were reported.[61] Taken together, laser-assisted minoxidil therapy is promising in the treatment of AGA, but larger studies are still needed.

LADD using a 1550-nm erbium-glass laser with minoxidil 5% in AA has been described in a single case series of 8 patients with patchy disease in adults and a child with AU.[62] Patients with patchy disease had evidence of hair regrowth, but the child with universalis did not have appreciable hair regrowth. Furthermore, the relapsing-remitting course of disease in AA makes objective assessment of long-standing hair regrowth difficult.

Although the use of minoxidil with LADD is encouraging, additional research is needed to bring this therapy to standard of care. Future research efforts focusing on the basic pharmacokinetic profile of LADD of minoxidil in combination with blinded randomized control trials are needed to evaluate safety and efficacy.

Finasteride

Finasteride, an effective oral medication in the treatment of AGA, can have significant side effects, including decreased libido and erectile dysfunction, making enhanced delivery of topical preparations an area of interest. A single case series investigating 1550-nm fractional erbium-glass laser-assisted delivery of finasteride 0.05% solution and an unspecified growth factor solution involving 4 patients with AGA led to a positive response in all patients by physician and patient assessment of global scalp photography.[63] The case series showed that topical finasteride may be a feasible treatment in AGA, but further studies are needed given the limited evidence.

Preliminary findings from a prospective trial reported use of 1550-nm fractional erbium glass laser in-assisted delivery of topical finasteride, biotin, and dexpanthenol led to increased hair density and growth in 100 patients with AGA.[64] However, the concomitant use of other topical agents prevents a definitive determination about the efficacy of topical finasteride. Similar to LADD of minoxidil, future studies are needed to determine the safety and efficacy of LADD of finasteride for AGA.

Corticosteroids

LADD of corticosteroids for treatment-resistant AA is an active area of research. A single study investigating 10 sessions of fractional CO_2-assisted delivery of triamcinolone solution (10 mg/mL) spaced 2 weeks apart in 10 patients with resistant AA reported 75% regrowth in all 8 subjects that completed at least 3 treatments.[65] One patient with AA of the beard received 3 split-face treatments and achieved a complete response only on the treated side. No adverse effects were reported.

A case series examining CO_2 and ultrasonography-assisted triamcinolone delivery for patients with treatment-resistant AA reported improvement in all patients after a single treatment.[66] A single patient who underwent laser-assisted delivery of triamcinolone without the use of ultrasonography on a single occipital patch only experienced minimal hair regrowth after 1 session, underscoring how ultrasonography can be used to further LADD treatment response. Larger-scale trials examining use of LADD of corticosteroids in AA are needed. Furthermore, use of ultrasonography with LADD has the potential for a synergistic treatment effect, which requires further study.

Limitations and Future Directions

Most studies examining LADD in the treatment of hair loss are small, preliminary feasibility trials. Future research including investigator-blinded randomized control trials are needed to advance the field. Patient safety and cost need to be addressed. Profiling the systemic absorption of various topical drugs delivered with laser assistance is necessary to anticipate treatment side effects. Laser therapy is not covered by insurance and is costly out of pocket. Insurance coverage, safety determination studies, and large-scale research trials examining treatment efficacy are underway and essential to advance the field.

RADIOFREQUENCY THERAPY

RF devices generate high-frequency electric currents. The molecular oscillation caused by the resistance of RF energy passing through human tissue generates thermal energy that has various therapeutic applications.[67] RF devices can be either monopolar or bipolar. Monopolar RF devices direct RF energy through a transducer in contact with the treatment area and use a ground pad on the patient's body.[68] In contrast, bipolar RF devices have electrodes spaced in close proximity and pass current through a narrow treatment zone, including microneedling devices equipped with insulated RF microneedles.[33] RF has been best studied in the use of skin rejuvenation and acne scar revision. However, a few studies have examined the use of RF devices in the treatment of hair loss.

An open-label study of RF in 25 patients with AGA showed a 31.6% increase in hair count and an 18% increase in hair thickness after 10 treatments at 2-week intervals.[69] No patients reported pain during the procedure and no adverse events were reported. However, hair counts and thickness were only evaluated in 10 of the patients treated. Similar encouraging results were reported in a blinded sham-device–controlled study in 24 men with AGA who received 4 RF treatments to affected scalp 3 weeks apart.[70]

Microneedling devices equipped with bipolar RF are thought to stimulate hair growth through both mechanical and thermal injury. A split-scalp study comparing 5 sessions of RF microneedling and postprocedural minoxidil with minoxidil monotherapy reported that combination therapy led to greater hair density and diameter than minoxidil monotherapy in 19 men with AGA.[33] Another-assisted drug delivery study reported resolution of patchy AA in 2 patients after several treatments of RF microneedle–assisted corticosteroid delivery.[71]

Limitations and Future Directions

RF technology uses a different mechanism of action than light-based devices to stimulate hair growth. RF has been reported to cause fewer pigmentary changes in people with darker skin types than light-based devices and can be adapted for combination treatment with multiple energy modalities.[1] However, more studies are needed to determine the safety and efficacy of RF as a treatment of hair and scalp disorders.

Summary

Energy-based devices are an emerging treatment option for hair loss. The scope of evidence supporting the use of energy-based devices in hair loss is limited, but existing studies potentiate their promise. Their safety and efficacy have primarily been evaluated in pattern hair loss. However, some energy-based devices have been investigated as treatments for reversible inflammatory and irreversible scarring hair disorders. Although the proposed mechanisms of action of these devices range from microscopic wounding to modulation of mitochondrial respiration, they share a favorable side effect profile. Energy-based devices are also united by a high cost of use and lack of insurance coverage, which has the potential to limit access. However, continued quality research increases the likelihood of large-scale manufacturing, decreased cost, and widespread insurance coverage. Despite key challenges, there is continued and growing excitement about the use of energy-based devices for hair loss.

CLINICS CARE POINTS

- Photobiomodulation devices (PBM) are available with and without hair-parting teeth. For those with mild to moderate hair density, recommend a PBM device with hair-parting teeth to ensure the low-level laser light reaches the scalp and is not absorbed or scattered by scalp hair.
- Patients using both topical alopecia medications and photobiomodulation (PBM) devices should be counseled to first treat dry scalp with PBM before application of topicals to prevent absorption and scattering of low-level laser light by topical medication.
- Photobiomodulation devices with many laser diodes are generally more expensive but require less active treatment time than those with fewer laser diodes.
- Patients interested in using a microneedling device should be counseled to select a device with microneedles 1.5 mm in length.
- Patients interested in fractionated laser therapy for treatment of alopecia should be counseled that there is limited evidence for the treatment and to only receive laser treatment from a trained professional, as there is a risk of ablating the hair follicle.
- There is limited data regarding the systemic absorption of topical drugs delivered with assistance from energy-based devices. Device-assisted drug delivery should be performed after careful screening and may require in-clinic monitoring for possible systemic side effects of topical medications delivered.

DISCLOSURE

The authors have nothing to disclose.

REFERENCES

1. Mester E, Szende B, Tota JG. Effect of laser on hair growth in mice. Kiserl Orvostud 1967;19:628–31.
2. Mester E, Szende B, Gartner P. The effect of laser beams on the growth of hair in mice. Radiobiol Radiother (Berl) 1968;9(5):621–6.
3. American Society for Laser Medicine & Surgery. Photobiomodulation. 2016. Available at: https://www.aslms.org/for-the-public/treatments-using-lasers-and-energy-based-devices/photobiomodulation. Accessed July 6, 2020.
4. Hamblin MR. Photobiomodulation for the management of alopecia: mechanisms of action, patient selection and perspectives. Clin Cosmet Investig Dermatol 2019;12:669–78.
5. Karu TI. Multiple roles of cytochrome c oxidase in mammalian cells under action of red and IR-A radiation. IUBMB Life 2010;62(8):607–10. https://doi.org/10.1002/iub.359.
6. Poyton RO, Ball KA. Therapeutic photobiomodulation: nitric oxide and a novel function of mitochondrial cytochrome c oxidase. Discov Med 2011;11(57):154–9.
7. Gupta AK, Bamimore MA, Foley KA. Efficacy of nonsurgical treatments for androgenetic alopecia in men and women: a systematic review with network meta-analyses, and an assessment of evidence quality. J Dermatol Treat 2020.
8. Leavitt M, Charles G, Heyman E, et al. HairMax LaserComb laser phototherapy device in the treatment of male androgenetic alopecia: a randomized, double-blind, sham device- controlled, multicentre trial. Clin Drug Investig 2009;29(5):283–92.
9. Avci P, Gupta A, Sadasivam M, et al. Low-level laser (light) therapy (LLLT) in skin: stimulating, healing, restoring. Semin Cutan Med Surg 2013;32(1):41–52.
10. Revian. Available at: https://revian.com/clinical-results/. Accessed July 6, 2020.
11. Sobanko JF, Alster TS. Efficacy of low-level laser therapy for chronic cutaneous ulceration in humans: a review and discussion. Dermatol Surg 2008;34(8):991–1000.
12. HairMax. Available at: http://www.Hairmax.Com. Accessed July 6, 2020.
13. Jimenez JJ, Wikramanayake TC, Bergfeld W, et al. Efficacy and safety of a low-level laser device in the treatment of male and female pattern hair loss: a multicenter, randomized, sham device-controlled, double-blind study. Am J Clin Dermatol 2014;15(2):115–27.
14. Satino JL, Markou M. Hair regrowth and increased hair tensile strength using the HairMax LaserComb for low-level laser therapy. Int J Cosmet Surg Aesthet Dermatol 2003;5(2).
15. Lanzafame RJ, Blanch RR, Bodian AB, et al. The growth of human scalp hair mediated by visible red light laser and LED sources in males. Lasers Surg Med 2013;45(8):487–95.
16. Lanzafame RJ, Blanche RR, Chiacchierini RP, et al. The growth of human scalp hair in females using visible red light laser and LED sources. Lasers Surg Med 2014;46(8):601–7.
17. Friedman S, Schnoor P. Novel approach to treating androgenetic alopecia in females with photobiomodulation (low-level laser therapy). Dermatol Surg 2017;43(6):856–67.
18. REV-01 Data on File. A multicenter, double-blind, placebo controlled study REVIAN RED cap or a Placebo Cap (no red light) ClinicalTrials.gov Identifier: NCT04019795.
19. Kim H, Choi JW, Kim JY, et al. Low-Level Light Therapy for androgenetic alopecia: a 24-week, randomized,

double-blind, sham device–controlled multicenter trial. Dermatol Surg 2013;39(8):1177–83.

20. Avram MR, Rogers NE. The use of low-level light for hair growth: part I. J Cosmet Laser Ther 2009;11(2):110–7.

21. Egger S, Resnik SR, Aickara D, et al. Examining the safety and efficacy of low-level laser therapy for male and female pattern hair loss: a review of the literature. Skin Appendage Disord 2020. https://doi.org/10.1159/000509001.

22. Fonda-Pascual P, Moreno-Arrones OM, Saceda-Corralo D, et al. Effectiveness of low-level laser therapy in lichen planopilaris. J Am Acad Dermatol 2018;78(5):1020–3.

23. Gerkowicz A, Bartosińska J, Wolska-Gawron K, et al. Application of superluminescent diodes (sLED) in the treatment of scarring alopecia: a pilot study. Photodiagnosis Photodyn Ther 2019;28:195–200.

24. Randolph MJ, Salhi WA, Tosti A. Lichen planopilaris and low-level light therapy: four case reports and review of the literature about low-level light therapy and lichenoid dermatosis. Dermatol Ther (Heidelb) 2020;10:311–9.

25. Fakhraei Lahiji S, Seo SH, Kim S, et al. Transcutaneous implantation of valproic acid-encapsulated dissolving microneedles induces hair regrowth. Biomaterials 2018. https://doi.org/10.1016/j.biomaterials.2018.03.019.

26. Serrano G, Almudéver P, Serrano JM, et al. Microneedling dilates the follicular infundibulum and increases transfollicular absorption of liposomal sepia melanin. Clin Cosmet Investig Dermatol 2015. https://doi.org/10.2147/CCID.S77228.

27. Fernandes D. Minimally invasive percutaneous collagen induction. Oral Maxillofac Surg Clin North Am 2005. https://doi.org/10.1016/j.coms.2004.09.004.

28. Doddaballapur S. Microneedling with dermaroller. J Cutan Aesthet Surg 2009. https://doi.org/10.4103/0974-2077.58529.

29. Bahuguna A. Micro needling - Facts and Fictions. Asian J Med Sci 2013. https://doi.org/10.3126/ajms.v4i3.5392.

30. Kim YS, Jeong KH, Kim JE, et al. Repeated microneedle stimulation induces enhanced hair growth in a murine model. Ann Dermatol 2016. https://doi.org/10.5021/ad.2016.28.5.586.

31. Starace M, Alessandrini A, Brandi N, Piraccini BM. Preliminary results of the use of scalp microneedling in different types of alopecia. J Cosmet Dermatol 2020;19(3):646–50. https://doi.org/10.1111/jocd.13061.

32. Dhurat R, Mathapati S. Response to microneedling treatment in men with androgenetic alopecia who failed to respond to conventional therapy. Indian J Dermatol 2015. https://doi.org/10.4103/0019-5154.156361.

33. Yu A-J, Luo Y-J, Xu X-G, et al. A pilot split-scalp study of combined fractional radiofrequency microneedling and 5% topical minoxidil in treating male pattern hair loss. Clin Exp Dermatol 2018;43(7):775–81. https://doi.org/10.1111/ced.13551.

34. Elias PM, Menon GK. Structural and lipid biochemical correlates of the epidermal permeability barrier. Adv Lipid Res 1991;24:1–26.

35. Eller MG, Szpunar GJ, Della-Coletta AA. Absorption of minoxidil after topical application: Effect of frequency and site of application. Clinical Pharmacology & Therapeutics 1989;45(4):396–402.

36. Choi N, Shin S, Song S, Sung J-H. Minoxidil Promotes Hair Growth through Stimulation of Growth Factor Release from Adipose-Derived Stem Cells. IJMS 2018;19(3):691. https://doi.org/10.3390/ijms19030691.

37. Deepak S, Shwetha S. Scalp roller therapy in resistant alopecia areata. J Cutan Aesthet Surg 2014. https://doi.org/10.4103/0974-2077.129988.

38. Mysore V, Chandrashekar B, Yepuri V. Alopecia areata-successful outcome with microneedling and triamcinolone acetonide. J Cutan Aesthet Surg 2014. https://doi.org/10.4103/0974-2077.129989.

39. Yoo KH, Lee JW, Li K, et al. Photodynamic therapy with methyl 5-aminolevulinate acid might be ineffective in recalcitrant alopecia totalis regardless of using a microneedle roller to increase skin penetration. Dermatol Surg 2010. https://doi.org/10.1111/j.1524-4725.2010.01515.x.

40. Dhurat R, Sukesh M, Avhad G, et al. A randomized evaluator blinded study of effect of microneedling in androgenetic alopecia: a pilot study. Int J Trichology 2013. https://doi.org/10.4103/0974-7753.114700.

41. Bao L, Gong L, Guo M, et al. Randomized trial of electrodynamic microneedle combined with 5% minoxidil topical solution for the treatment of Chinese male Androgenetic alopecia. J Cosmet Laser Ther 2020;22(1):1–7. https://doi.org/10.1080/14764172.2017.1376094.

42. Nilforooshzadeh MA, Lotfi E, Heidari-Kharaji M, Zolghadr S, Mansouri P. Effective combination therapy with high concentration of Minoxidil and Carboxygas in resistant Androgenetic alopecia: Report of nine cases. J Cosmet Dermatol 2020;19(11):2953–7. https://doi.org/10.1111/jocd.13362.

43. Shah KB, Shah AN, Solanki RB, et al. A comparative study of microneedling with platelet-rich plasma plus topical minoxidil (5%) and topical minoxidil (5%) alone in androgenetic alopecia. Int J Trichology 2017. https://doi.org/10.4103/ijt.ijt_75_16.

44. Jha AK, Udayan UK, Roy PK, et al. Original article: Platelet-rich plasma with microneedling in androgenetic alopecia along with dermoscopic pre- and post-treatment evaluation. J Cosmet Dermatol 2018. https://doi.org/10.1111/jocd.12394.

45. Breedis C. Regeneration of hair follicles and sebaceous glands from the epithelium of scars in the rabbit. Cancer Res 1954;14:575–9.

46. Avram M, Hruza G. Lasers and lights: procedures in cosmetic dermatology. Amsterdam, Netherlands: Elsevier Health Sciences; 2013.

47. Ke J, Guan H, Li S, et al. YAG laser (2,940 nm) treatment stimulates hair growth through upregulating Wnt 10b and β-catenin expression in C57BL/6 mice 2015;8(11):20883–9.

48. Lee G-Y, Lee S-J, Kim W-S. The effect of a 1550 nm fractional erbium-glass laser in female pattern hair loss: Fractional photothermolysis laser treatment of female pattern hair loss. J Eur Acad Dermatol Venereol 2011;25(12):1450–4.

49. Cho SB, Goo BL, Zheng Z, et al. Therapeutic efficacy and safety of a 1927-nm fractionated thulium laser on pattern hair loss: an evaluator-blinded, split-scalp study. Lasers Med Sci 2018;33(4):851–9.

50. Bahrani E, Lauw MIS, Tabatabai ZL, et al. Letters and Communications. Dermatologic Surgery.4.

51. Eckert MM, Gundin NL, Crespo RL. Alopecia areata: good response to treatment with fractional laser in 5 cases. J Cosmo Trichol 2016;2(2).

52. Alhattab MK, AL Abdullah MJ, Al-janabi MH, et al. The effect of 1540-nm fractional erbium-glass laser in the treatment of androgenic alopecia. J Cosmet Dermatol 2020;19(4):878–83.

53. Cho S, Choi MJ, Zheng Z, et al. Clinical effects of non-ablative and ablative fractional lasers on various hair disorders: a case series of 17 patients. J Cosmet Laser Ther 2013;15(2):74–9.

54. Alopecia areata treated with fractional photothermolysis laser: a case report. J Am Acad Dermatol 2016; 74(5):AB132.

55. Yoo KH, Kim MN, Kim BJ, et al. Treatment of alopecia areata with fractional photothermolysis laser. Int J Dermatol 2009. https://doi.org/10.1111/j.1365-4632.2009.04230.x.

56. Yalici-Armagan B, Elcin G. The effect of neodymium: yttrium aluminum garnet and fractional carbon dioxide lasers on alopecia areata. Dermatol Surg 2016; 42(4):500–6.

57. Haedersdal M, Erlendsson AM, Paasch U, et al. Translational medicine in the field of ablative fractional laser (AFXL)-assisted drug delivery: a critical review from basics to current clinical status. J Am Acad Dermatol 2016;74(5):981–1004.

58. ClinicalTrials.gov [Internet]. Identifier NCT03852992, Laser Assisted Delivery of Minoxidil in Androgenetic Alopecia. Bethesda (MD): National Library of Medicine (US); 2019. Available at: https://clinicaltrials.gov/ct2/show/NCT03852992. Clinical Trials.gov. Accessed August 2020, 11.

59. Lee W, Shen S, Aljuffali IA, et al. Erbium–Yttrium–Aluminum–Garnet Laser irradiation ameliorates skin permeation and follicular delivery of antialopecia drugs. J Pharm Sci 2014;103(11):3542–52.

60. Salah M, Samy N, Fawzy MM, et al. The effect of the fractional carbon dioxide laser on improving minoxidil delivery for the treatment of androgenetic alopecia. J Lasers Med Sci 2019;11(1):29–36.

61. Suchonwanit P, Rojhirunsakool S, Khunkhet S. A randomized, investigator-blinded, controlled, split-scalp study of the efficacy and safety of a 1550-nm fractional erbium-glass laser, used in combination with topical 5% minoxidil versus 5% minoxidil alone, for the treatment of androgenetic alopecia. Lasers Med Sci 2019;34(9):1857–64.

62. Wang W, Gegentana, Tonglaga, et al. Treatment of alopecia areata with nonablative fractional laser combined with topical minoxidil. J Cosmet Dermatol 2019;18(4):1009–13.

63. Bertin ACJ, Vilarinho A, Junqueira ALA. Fractional non-ablative laser-assisted drug delivery leads to improvement in male and female pattern hair loss. J Cosmet Laser Ther 2018;20(7–8):391–4.

64. Marques E, Almeida F, Almeida L, et al, A 48 month clinical follow up of female and male pattern hair loss treatment with a one month fractional laser and transepidermal drug delivery session in 100 Brazilian patients. 36th Annual Conference of the American Society for laser medicine and surgery, Boston, MA: Conference Publication, 2016;48:7–8.

65. Majid I, Jeelani S, Imran S. Fractional carbon dioxide laser in combination with topical corticosteroid application in resistant alopecia areata: a case series. J Cutan Aesthet Surg 2018;11(4):217.

66. Issa MCA, Pires M, Silveira P, et al. Transepidermal drug delivery: a new treatment option for areata alopecia? J Cosmet Laser Ther 2015;17(1):37–40.

67. Mulholland RS. Radio frequency energy for non-invasive and minimally invasive skin tightening. Clin Plast Surg 2011;38(3):437–48.

68. Carruthers J, Fabi S, Weiss R. Monopolar radiofrequency for skin tightening: our experience and a review of the literature. Dermatol Surg 2014;40:S168–73.

69. Verner I, Lotti T. Clinical evaluation of a novel fractional radiofrequency device for hair growth: fractional radiofrequency for hair growth stimulation. Dermatol Ther 2018;31(3):e12590.

70. Tan Y, Wei L, Zhang Y, et al. Non-ablative radio frequency for the treatment of androgenetic alopecia. Acta Dermatovenerol Alp Pannonica Adriat 2019;28(4):169–71.

71. Issa MCA, Pires M, Silveira P, Xavier de Brito E, Sasajima C. Transepidermal drug delivery: A new treatment option for areata alopecia? Journal of Cosmetic and Laser Therapy 2015;17(1):37–40. https://doi.org/10.3109/14764172.2014.967778.

72. Tsai, et al. Alopecia areata treated with fractional photothermolysis laser: A case report. Journal of the American Academy of Dermatology 2016; 74(5):AB132-AB132.

73. Mendieta-Eckert M, Landa-Gundin N, Torrontegui-Bilbao J. Treatment of Patchy and Universalis Alopecia Areata With Fractional Laser. Dermatol Surg 2020;46(3):430–3.

Hair Transplantation and Follicular Unit Extraction

Kristina Collins, MD[a],*, Marc R. Avram, MD[a,b]

KEYWORDS

- Hair transplantation • FUE • Alopecia • Hair loss

KEY POINTS

- Hair transplantation procedures have evolved throughout the years to produce consistently natural results.
- Patient preoperative evaluation and management of expectations is extremely important.
- Preoperative and postoperative medical management of hair loss improves long-term results.
- The surgeon needs to use an artistic eye to plan the transplant considering the likely long-term trajectory of hair loss.
- The surgeon plans to use strip harvesting versus follicular unit extraction (FUE) based on patient characteristics; FUE can be accomplished manually, with machine assistance, or with an automated robotic device.

INTRODUCTION/BACKGROUND/PREVALENCE

Hair loss affects both men and women and, for many people, profoundly impacts psychosocial function and psychological well-being.[1] Few other physical signs of aging demonstrate such direct correlation with self-esteem and self-worth. Hair has long been associated with youth, vitality, and health; and our individual hair styles frame our faces and communicate information about our unique personalities. Given our subconscious and conscious perceptions about hair, it is not surprising that involuntary hair loss frequently provokes emotional distress.[2,3] Fortunately for our patients, medical and surgical treatment options can stop their hair loss and often reverse the physical signs of hair loss Today, follicular unit hair transplantation (FUT) and follicular unit extraction (FUE) provide the surgeon with incredible versatility in terms of graft placement and design, leading to consistent and natural cosmetic results.

The history of hair transplantation dates back to Japan in the 1930s where physicians experimented with using dermal punch grafts from the scalp to transplant hair onto scarred areas of alopecia on the scalp, eyebrows, or other parts of the body.[4,5] In New York in the 1950s, a dermatologist named Dr Norman Orentreich began experimenting with large punch grafts from the posterior and lateral scalp to the areas of the scalp affected by androgenetic alopecia and demonstrated the fundamental mechanism of hair transplantation, the principle of donor dominance, which observes that hair follicle grafts continue to match the growth characteristics of the donor site even after transplantation to a recipient site. These initial grafts were 2 to 4 mm in size and had 15 to 30 follicular units in each one.[6] Hair transplantation was a scientific success but often a cosmetic failure. The reason was the size of the grafts used with multiple follicular units in each graft. It looked unnatural because it was unnatural. Hair on our scalp grows in individual 1-hair to 4-hair follicular units. Beginning in the early 1990s, the size of individual grafts began shrinking to the point that individual follicular units became the standard size graft used in the procedure. This evolution has led to consistently naturally appearing transplanted hair

[a] Private Practice, Austin Skin, 15601 SH 71 West Suite 200, Austin, TX 78738, USA; [b] Weill Cornell Medical School, New York, NY, USA
* Corresponding author.
E-mail address: kristina.m.collins@gmail.com

Dermatol Clin 39 (2021) 463–478
https://doi.org/10.1016/j.det.2021.04.003

for our patients.[7–9] Patients over the past 20 years have benefited from surgeon's ability to create natural-appearing transplanted hair (**Figs. 1** and **2**).

Harvesting the donor grafts is performed by either elliptical excision of a horizontal strip (FUT) or by removal of individual follicular groupings from the posterior scalp with a 0.75-mm to 1.2-mm punch device (**Fig. 3**). Both of these techniques have advantages and disadvantages that dictate the best plan for each patient. Notably, the short trimming of hair necessary for FUE is not acceptable for most patients with long hair styles, and harvesting the grafts from a well-concealed strip is preferable in those cases. Compared with FUT, FUE is less labor intensive in terms of graft preparation, minimizes postoperative recovery; decreases risk of bleeding, nerve injury, visible scarring, or other complications; and can be used in cases with tight scalp skin or in body hair transplantation. However, FUE has a longer learning curve, higher transection rate of follicles, a wider donor area, and longer procedure duration. Both FUT and FUE provide excellent cosmetic results for properly selected patients.[10–12] This article focuses on the preoperative and preoperative management of patients presenting for FUE as well as discuss the procedural steps in detail (**Table 1**).

PATIENT EVALUATION OVERVIEW

A thorough patient evaluation and an understanding of the pathophysiology of hair loss are essential components to successful hair transplantation. Although individuals of all skin types and all hair colors can be candidates for hair restoration, factors such as hair follicle density, average caliber of hair shaft, pattern of alopecia, and age of the patient all play vital roles in patient selection

and operative planning.[13] The surgeon uses the clinical history of hair loss, the predicted pattern of future loss, and the physical examination of the follicles and shafts of hair to anticipate the treatment course and set realistic patient expectations. Physicians must anticipate future hair loss when designing their hair transplant.[14] The plan should be for natural-appearing transplanted hair 1 year and 10 years after the procedure (**Fig. 4**).

The vast majority of hair transplant patients present with hair loss secondary to male or female pattern hair loss. Hair thinning and eventually hair loss occurs due to progressive miniaturization of genetically predisposed follicles in predictable regions of the frontal and vertex scalp along with a rise in the telogen/anagen ratio of follicles in these zones. Physical examination determining androgenetic alopecia is usually straightforward; however, if any areas of scarring, bogginess, inflammation, or follicular plugging are noted on physical examination, a scalp biopsy may be indicated to determine an underlying cause of alopecia that may respond to medical management of an inflammatory condition. If a patient has an active inflammatory scalp condition, hair transplantation is not an option until the skin disease is medically managed.[14,15]

The history of hair loss is also important and a more extensive workup is appropriate if onset occurred within 1 year. Certain hair styles contribute to hair loss, including bleaching, straightening, extensions, wigs/hairpieces, or tightly woven braids. Medications and supplements, including isotretinoin, acitretin, beta blockers, ACE inhibitors, selenium, high doses of vitamin A, antidepressants, cholesterol medications, warfarin, and chemotherapeutics, can contribute to hair thinning. Telogen effluvium due to stress, illness, or childbirth leads to pronounced yet reversible changes in hair density.[16–19] Genetic

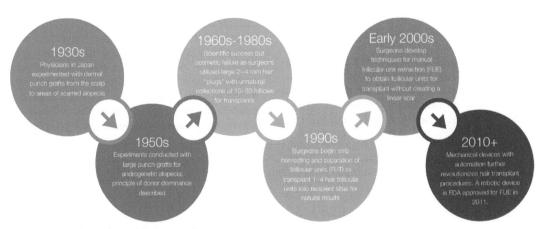

Fig. 1. Historical timeline of hair transplants.

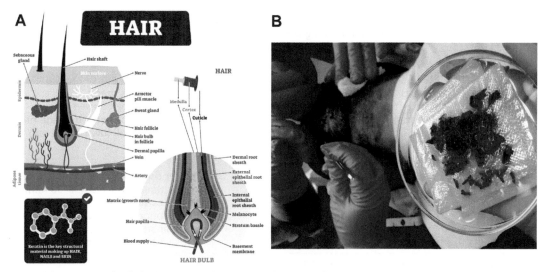

Fig. 2. (*A*) Diagram of a follicular unit and anatomy of the hair follicle. (*B*) Follicular units in saline. ([*A*] With permission from Shutterstock Inc.; and [*B*] *Courtesy of* M. Avram, MD, New York, New York.)

factors play a major role in hair loss, and family history is useful in evaluation of the patient and anticipating the future clinical outcome. However, male and female hair loss is polygenic with contribution from both maternal and paternal genes, so even a detailed family history fails to accurately predict the clinical course for each individual patient.

Overall for men, the androgen receptor (AR) gene on the X chromosome appears to be the main genetic determinant of hair loss.[20,21]

Female patients in particular present with a number of diagnostic variables that require further evaluation. Hormonal fluctuations due to menopause, birth control, childbirth, or polycystic ovary

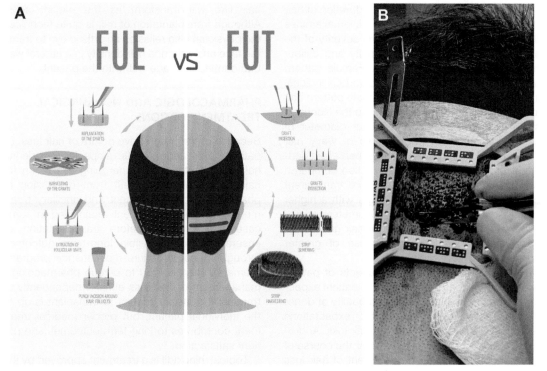

Fig. 3. (*A*) Pictorial of strip harvesting (FUT) versus follicular unit extraction (FUE). (*B*) Clinical photo of FUE donor site. ([*A*] With permission from Shutterstock Inc.; and [*B*] *Courtesy of* M. Avram, MD, New York, New York.)

Table 1
Pros and cons to consider when determining whether to use FUT or FUE

Technique	Pros	Cons
FUT	• Minimal risk of transection of hair follicles • Shorter time to harvest (10–20 min) • Hair does not have to be trimmed and scar is usually easily hidden within hair • Usually no visible scar	• Visible scar with short hair; More work to prepare grafts • Body hair cannot be used • Higher chance of nerve damage or bleeding (but still low risk overall)
FUE	• Minimal graft preparation; body hair can be used; potential to incorporate automation and greater use of technology; minimally invasive • Can be done for patients with tight scalps	• Greater risk of transection of follicles • Longer time to harvest (30–90 min); longer learning curve • Wider donor area required; hair must be trimmed short (not ideal for patients with long hair styles)

Abbreviations: FUE, follicular unit extraction; FUT, follicular unit transplantation.
[a]Both FUT and FUE provide excellent cosmetic results but the pros and cons of each procedure can help determine the best plan of action for the individual patient.

syndrome should be considered in the pathophysiology of hair loss in a female patient. Thyroid levels, vitamin D levels, and ferritin levels should generally be obtained in women presenting with new-onset hair loss as appropriate medical management of these abnormalities is essential to slowing the progression of alopecia and regaining control of hair growth in these patients[16,18] (**Fig. 5**).

Once a clinical background and duration of hair loss have been reviewed, the physician examines the pattern of thinning, grades the severity of the alopecia, and evaluates the density and caliber of hair follicles and hair shafts. Female pattern hair loss[22] is graded according to various indices, including the Ludwig Scale, and male pattern hair loss is typically graded according to the Norwood scale (**Fig. 6**). Patients with higher diameter of hairs, such as those with coarse or wavy hair (>80 μm of shaft), will see a greater *perceived* density improvement after transplantation compared with patients with very fine or more transparent hair (<60 μm). In addition, patients with a higher number of follicles per square centimeter and patients with a larger donor area of hair growth will have improved outcomes because of greater numbers of follicles to harvest.[23–25]

One of the most important aspects of patient evaluation includes management of patient expectations based on the amount and quality of donor hair available as well as realistic expectations regarding the pattern of ongoing hair loss. Androgenetic alopecia is progressive over the course of an individual's life and the treatment of hair loss needs to be ongoing as well. Furthermore, the transplant must be planned according to the anticipated future pattern of loss for the patient. For example, if a young man receives a transplant of hair in the vertex of the scalp, expanding hair loss on the lateral and posterior scalp as the patient ages can lead to an unnatural island of hair at the vertex. In general, hair transplanted on the frontal scalp retains a natural look over time as long as consideration is given to how the anterior hair line will transform as the patient ages. Although transplantation of hair is quite technical, the physician also relies on an artistic eye to frame the face and enhance hair density in a natural way that continues to age well with the patient.

PHARMACOLOGIC AND NONSURGICAL TREATMENT OPTIONS

Because of the progressive nature of hair loss, all patients with androgenetic alopecia considering hair transplantation or undergoing evaluation for hair transplantation benefit from discussion of pharmacologic management and ancillary treatments that help the patient retain, and in some cases, regrow hair before transplantation or ensure the best possible long-term outcomes through a postprocedure maintenance program. Ultimately the decision to pursue pharmacologic management of hair loss either independently of transplant or as an adjunct to transplant is up to the individual patient, but proper medical treatment contributes to long-term outcomes and patient satisfaction.

Topical minoxidil is a treatment approved by the Food and Drug Administration for male and female pattern hair loss. The direct mechanism of action

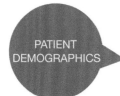

PATIENT DEMOGRAPHICS

All ages, all skin types, and both genders are appropriate candidates for hair transplantation. In younger patients, anticipation of the future progression of hair loss is paramount. Female hair loss may require more extensive work-up. The surgeon needs to be aware of unique challenges in transplantation of afrocentric hair.

CLINICAL HISTORY

Hair loss of less than one year duration requires more extensive evaluation. Medical history and medication lists should be checked to determine any exacerbating factors for hair loss.

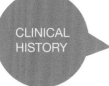

PHYSICAL EXAM

Androgenetic alopecia is usually straightforward on exam. Scalp should be examined for any signs of inflammatory disease or other form of alopecia, either scarring or non-scarring. Erythema, scale, follicular plugging, or bogginess are signs of inflammatory disease. Scalp elasticity and any signs of past surgery or scars should be noted for surgical planning. The pattern of thinning and grade of alopecia are observed (Norwood and Ludwig scales).

CALIBER OF HAIR FOLLICLES

Patients with a larger diameter of the hair shaft (ie- coarse/wavy hair, >80 microns) will see a greater perceived density after transplant compared to those with fine hair (<60 microns)

DONOR DENSITY AND HAIR DENSITY

Patients with a higher number of follicles per square centimeter and larger donor area of hair growth are better candidates. Patients with a larger number of hairs in each follicular unit (3-4 vs 1-2 hairs) have better outcomes.

PREVIOUS HAIR LOSS TREATMENTS

All other attempted hair loss treatments and the duration of treatments should be discussed. Ideally hair transplant candidates utilize medication management, PRP, or red light therapy for hair loss for 6 months to a year prior to undergoing surgery. Due to the cyclic phases of hair growth it can take up to a year to fully evaluate treatment efficacy. These treatments should be continued after transplant. Inflammatory skin disease must be medically managed prior to surgery.

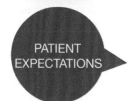

PATIENT EXPECTATIONS

A frank discussion needs to take place with the patient to inform them about their projected future hair loss and how this affects the surgical plan (for example, avoiding transplant to vertex for younger patients). The surgeon sets realistic expectations for the patient based on their hair caliber, density, and other physical exam elements..

Fig. 4. Evaluating a patient for hair transplant.

in hair growth is not fully understood, but its angiogenic and vasodilatory properties are thought to contribute. Daily use of minoxidil may increase the caliber of hair and also increase the duration of time follicles spend in the anagen (active growth) phase. The most bothersome side effect

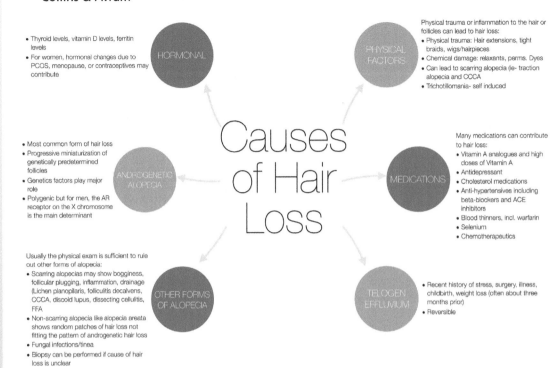

Fig. 5. Causes of hair loss. CCCA, central centrifugal cicatricial alopecia; FFA, frontal fibrosing alopecia; PCOS, polycystic ovary syndrome.

of the medication is unwanted hair growth on the face. Dizziness, palpitations, and short-term shedding of hair also may occur.[26–28]

Finasteride is FDA approved for treating male pattern baldness and acts by blockade of 5-alpha-reductase and reduction of dihydrotestosterone (DHT). Five-year results of a randomized study found that 90% of patients showed hair growth above baseline with finasteride 1 mg daily.[29] Although treatment of thinning of hair in the vertex is the approved indication, hair growth has also been shown to occur in the anterior scalp. Patients who continue finasteride after hair transplantation had greater hair counts at 48 weeks after surgery than in placebo groups. Overall, the drug is well tolerated but it does cause a predictable decrease in the prostate specific antigen; 2% to 5% of men report sexual side effects including decreased libido, erectile dysfunction, or reduction in fertility. Published trials show these sexual side effects are reversible if the finasteride is discontinued. However, there are reports of a condition called post finasteride syndrome, in which men experience persistent long-term sexual side effects or depression after cessation of finasteride treatment. The incidence of post finasteride syndrome is unknown. Patients should be made aware of this risk before beginning finasteride. Women of childbearing age should not use finasteride because of teratogenic effects.[30–37]

Low-level light therapy (or red light therapy) uses LED (light-emitting diode) lights in the 650-nm to 700-nm wavelength to increase circulation of the scalp and increase metabolism of the hair follicle. There are numerous red light combs and helmets on the market that prove useful as an adjunctive treatment, particularly for patients who have experienced side effects during pharmacologic management of hair loss.[38]

Platelet-rich plasma (PRP) is separated from the patient's own blood by centrifuge and contains densely packed platelets and growth factors. The fluid is injected directly into areas of hair thinning on the scalp in a series of 4 treatments spaced 1 month apart. Maintenance treatments twice yearly are encouraged. There are many recent clinical trials that confirm the efficacy of PRP in treating male and female pattern hair loss.[39]

Encouraging all of the preceding modalities at once would overwhelm most patients and lead to poor treatment adherence. It is the opinion of the author that patients with hair loss should be encouraged to be diligent with 2 of the preceding modalities long-term, depending on their specific patient characteristics and preferences. The surgeon needs to work with the patient to identify which treatment modalities best suit the patient's preferences so that they will partner in long-term management of the chronic condition of hair loss. Some patients prefer to avoid medication management altogether, and feel comfortable returning for further transplant

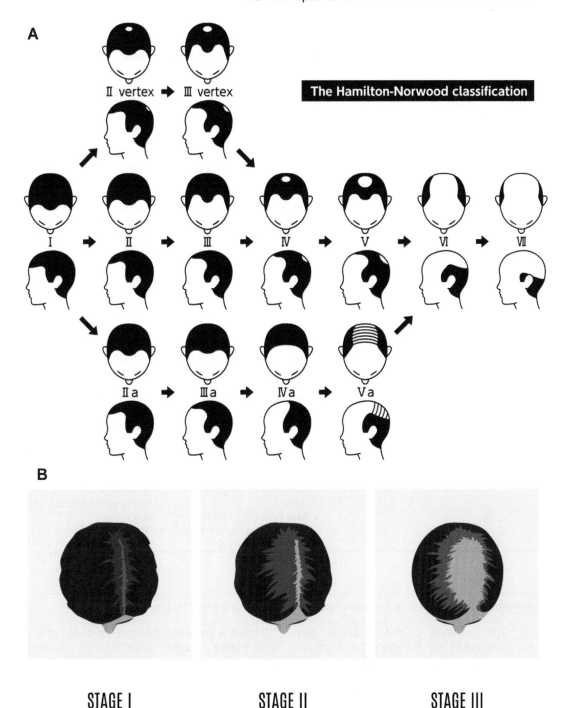

Fig. 6. (*A*) Norwood scale for male pattern baldness. (*B*). Ludwig scale for female pattern hair loss. (With permission from Shutterstock Inc.)

procedures as the hair thins; this is acceptable as long as the patient is well informed (**Table 2**).

SURGICAL/INTERVENTIONAL TREATMENT OPTIONS

Once the patient has undergone thorough evaluation, understands the long-term trajectory of hair loss, commits to a hair loss management plan, and decides to proceed with hair transplantation, operative planning begins. Hair transplantation involves a high degree of precision, technology integration, and utilization of an incredibly skilled surgical team, but also requires an abstract and artistic approach to recreate a style that appears

Table 2
Comparison of pros and cons of nonsurgical treatments for androgenetic alopecia

Medication	Mechanism of Action	Benefits	Adverse Effects/Cons
Minoxidil	Not fully understood: angiogenic and vasodilatory properties and role as a potassium channel opener may increase the caliber of hair and increase duration of anagen phase	• FDA approved for male and female pattern hair loss • Relatively safe and inexpensive • Helpful in the peri-transplant period for stabilizing existing hairs and shortening the time for transplanted hair to begin growing	• Unwanted hair growth on the face, dizziness, palpitations, and short-term shedding of hair may occur • Women with a tendency to grow dark facial hair may need to use the 2% solution • People with contact dermatitis to propylene glycol need to use the branded Rogaine 5% foam • Fetal hypertrichosis can occur when used by pregnant women
Finasteride	Blockade of 5-alpha reductase and reduction of dihydrotestosterone	• 1 mg dosage FDA approved for male pattern hair loss of the vertex in men • Studies also demonstrate hair regrowth in the anterior scalp • Use in combination with hair transplant surgery has shown greater hair counts postoperatively • Well-tolerated, easy, convenient, taken once daily • May help with hair loss in women at a higher dose (2.5 mg); not FDA approved	• Major teratogenic effects (feminizing a male fetus) • Caution in patients with liver disease, as the drug is metabolized by the liver • PCP must be informed because PSA levels decrease by half • 2%–5% of men report decreased libido, erectile dysfunction, or ejaculation issues • Rarely gynecomastia and depression • Post-finasteride syndrome: few reports of men with long-term effects after discontinuing treatment

Abbreviations: FDA, Food and Drug Administration; PCP, primary care provider; PSA, prostate-specific antigen.

natural. This marriage of detail-oriented and artistic components set the stage for a unique and rewarding procedure for the surgeon.

Hair transplantation is a lengthy procedure and requires a highly skilled and coordinated team usually consisting of the surgeon working alongside 2 to 5 surgical assistants. There is no specific certification program that creates an exceptional surgical assistant. Training of the hair transplantation team requires consistent focused effort. It is recommended that the physician learns the procedure alongside the assistant and that the transplant team starts with smaller surgeries (fewer than 300 grafts at first) to gain skill without being overwhelmed. The surgeon should anticipate that it will take 6 to 12 months and more than several dozen procedures before a surgical assistant feels completely prepared for large or complex cases. Overall, most hair transplantation procedures take the surgical team between 3 and 8 hours, with greater duration of surgery depending on the number of follicular units transplanted. An experienced team may transplant 1000 to 2500 grafts during a single procedure. In prepping for the procedure, standardization of photography of the hair and hair line is strongly recommended, with consistent lighting, patient positioning, and photograph background. In the description that follows, we briefly review the essentials of FUT and focus our discussion on procedural details for FUE.

FOLLICULAR UNIT TRANSPLANTATION

The first major step in preoperative planning is determining whether the patient will have FUT or FUE. The typical donor zone for FUT lies in a 5-cm to 6-cm wide horizontal band in the occipital scalp. The strip should lie above the nuchal ridge but not so high that ongoing recession of the lateral and posterior hairline may recede below the donor site with progressive hair loss as the patient ages, leading to a visible donor scar. We discussed preoperative evaluation of the patient as a candidate for hair transplantation with close examination of the patient's hair for caliber of the hair shafts (diameter of individual hairs), follicular unit density (number of follicular units per cm^2), and hair density (the number of hairs per cm^2). Patients with large-caliber hair shafts greater than 80 μm will achieve fuller coverage, likewise detection of early miniaturization of hair in the donor site helps to prevent a poor or unpredictable surgical outcome. As previously stated, good candidates for transplantation demonstrate follicular unit density of at least 40 FUs/cm but the surgeon also considers the follicular unit composition, or the pattern of natural hair groupings in the patient's follicular units, with a higher number of hairs per follicular unit more desirable.[11,40,41] Patients of Asian or African ethnicity frequently have a lower donor density than Caucasians, and it is essential to consider donor density challenges in decisions about the method of harvesting the hair and in the number of follicular units required. The formula to calculate the size of the donor strip needed is as follows:

> Number of follicular units desired to harvest = follicular unit density × area of donor strip (cm^2)

In evaluation of the donor site, the scalp elasticity of the patient requires consideration, especially if the surgeon plans to excise a strip with a width greater than 1.2 cm (typical width ranges from 0.8 to 1.2 cm).[42] The Mayer-Paul formula describes a method to determine scalp elasticity based on the distance the thumbs can compress scalp tissue between 2 dots marked at a distance 5 cm apart. The formula follows:

> (50 mm − new compressed distance between the 2 dots) × 100 = percent scalp elasticity

The ideal method for excising the strip aims to minimize damage to follicles with tension donor dissection. The edges of the strip are superficially scored with the scalpel and 2 skin hooks are placed on the outer edges of the incisions (or a "Haber Spreader" instrument is applied) to provide traction perpendicular to the wound. The remaining depth of the strip requires pressure and separation of the follicles without much cutting, minimizing transection of hair follicles. The strip extends down into the subcutaneous tissue, underneath the bulb of the hair follicles but more superficial than the deep vasculature. A trichophytic closure of the wound in which 1 to 2 mm of one wound edge is trimmed using sharp tip scissors before closure helps create a less noticeable scar.[43] Undermining of the wound and placement of dermal sutures are usually not necessary, and the choice between staples or epidermal sutures rests solely on personal preference of the surgeon. Most patients ultimately form a minimally visible, thin surgical scar at the donor site, but all patients require education about the possibility of poor wound healing with a wide scar or keloid formation. The hair transplant team uses optimal ergonomic positioning and magnification while separating 500 to 2000 follicular units from the strip in 1 to 3 hours. The follicles are prepped for grafting and placed into cool saline.

Follicular Unit Extraction

We now focus on the intricacies of FUE. For patients with short hair styles, this technique allows the surgeon to obtain a large number of grafts with little to no visible scarring using a 0.75-mm to 1.2-mm punch device. FUE can be performed manually, with device assistance, or with a fully automated robotic device. FUE involves a longer learning curve to overcome the higher risk of transection of follicles and longer procedure times. The development of FUE helped improve the popularity of the hair transplant procedure as the possibility of a relatively scarless procedure draws the interest of many potential patients. Importantly, FUE also set the foundation for incorporation of minimally invasive and automized technologies into the hair transplant procedure, modernizing our capabilities and improving outcomes.[10,44–46]

Patient Preparation and Anesthesia

On arrival, the team first trims the patient's hair in the donor region using electric razors to approximately 1 mm length. The surgeon marks the recipient site borders with an artistic eye, predicting future progression of hair loss and planning the ideal obtainable hairline for the patient. Surgical site preparation with chlorhexidine reduces the risk of infection.

Fortunately, patients tolerate the hair transplant procedure extremely well with local anesthesia. The lengthy nature of the procedure makes conscious sedation or general anesthesia nonpreferred options. In addition, prone patient positioning during the extraction of donor site grafts poses an airway risk for sedated patients. We recommend utilization of local anesthesia whenever possible to minimize unnecessary procedure risk. For sensitive or apprehensive patients, a low dose of an anxiolytic can be orally administered. Administration of lidocaine 1% with epinephrine into the dermis circumferentially around and throughout the donor site provides excellent anesthesia and hemostasis. In the recipient site, supratrochlear and supraorbital nerve blocks provide initial frontal scalp anesthesia and 1% lidocaine with epinephrine is directly injected into the recipient zone. Many surgeons also use the addition of 0.25% bupivacaine with epinephrine in the recipient zone for a longer duration of anesthesia.

There are many ways to support the patient during the administration of anesthesia and help reduce pain without increasing risk. Patients often feel more comfortable with distraction from the procedure; encourage patients to bring headphones to listen to music or a favorite podcast and allow them to look at their smartphone or a TV screen hanging above. The benefits of humor and conversation cannot be overstated in terms of comfort for some patients. Make an effort to develop an intuition about which patients prefer to "zone out" and listen to their headphones silently and which patients prefer to feel connected to the team with conversation. It is important to remember that during this long procedure the patient hears the team talking among each other. Make sure the conversations are calming and the noise in the room is not perceived as chaotic given the number of people present. All team members should resist statements like "oops" or "I'm sorry," as these can be misinterpreted by the patient to be related to an incident in their procedure. Remember that the patient also observes the operating room visually, and attempt to keep work areas clean and organized and minimize the opportunities for the patient to see bloody gauze on the tray or in the trash receptacle. Handheld vibrational devices held onto the patient's skin help reduce pain during injection. Always try to ensure the patient is as comfortable as possible in their position in the chair, especially in the prone position. They will need to hold the same prone position for a lengthy period of time, so check to make sure their neck is straight and their feet are comfortably placed on the ground. The patient should be placed in a comfortable reclined supine position for all other parts of the procedure, other than anesthesia and extraction of the donor area (**Fig. 7**).

Recipient Site Preparation

The most important element in achieving a natural looking hair transplant is planning of the anterior hairline.[45] For most male patients, the most anterior point of the hairline is in the midline 7.5 to 9.5 cm above the glabella. Many patients will be expected to continue experiencing gradual temporal hairline recession as well; therefore, most patients benefit from a higher placement of the hairline. Explain the hairline placement to the patient in detail in the mirror to manage expectations and help them visualize the likely future of their hairline. The ideal hairline demonstrates imperfect edges with a gradual transition to denser follicles posteriorly. The hairline should be feathered with irregular pattern follicles and not densely packed. Female patients generally do not need recreation of an anterior hairline but an increased density of their stable but thinning anterior hairline.

Many surgeons use #19-gauge or #20-gauge needles for preparation of the recipient sites. Careful attention to the existing hair is necessary to avoid transecting any existing hair follicles during recipient wound creation. The puncture wound should mimic the natural 30 to 45° angle of hair growth on the scalp. The sites should be placed in an irregular pattern with 10 to 30 sites per cm². The recipient site is frequently prepared before extraction of the donor grafts because of the decreased viability of grafts with longer duration of time before implantation. As previously stated, administration of bupivacaine after infiltration with lidocaine helps extend the duration of anesthesia of the recipient site.

Extraction of Grafts

The patient is placed in a prone position, and if robotic extraction is being performed, a specific chair is required for proper function of the device. It is possible to achieve excellent results using a handheld device but the speed of the surgical team will influence how many grafts can be obtained using this method. Motorized punches help improve speed and robotic devices improve both speed and angle accuracy.[47] The angle of the punch instrument during penetration must mimic the natural angle of hair as closely as possible to minimize transection of follicles. The grafts are placed in chilled 0.9% isotonic saline or in a variety of other holding solutions The grafts should never be allowed to get dry. FUE requires much less graft preparation than FUT. The donor sites are left to heal by secondary intention with minimal scarring for the vast majority of patients. Wound care consists of applying emollient to the

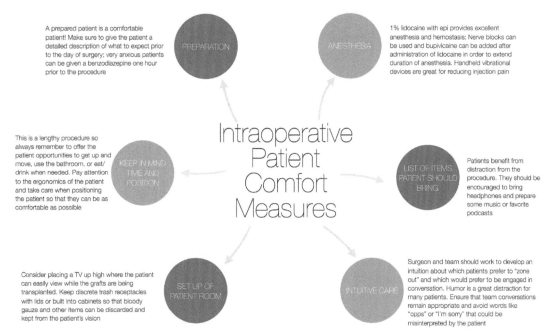

A prepared patient is a comfortable patient! Make sure to give the patient a detailed description of what to expect prior to the day of surgery; very anxious patients can be given a benzodiazepine one hour prior to the procedure

PREPARATION

ANESTHESIA

1% lidocaine with epi provides excellent anesthesia and hemostasis; Nerve blocks can be used and bupivicaine can be added after administration of lidocaine in order to extend duration of anesthesia. Handheld vibrational devices are great for reducing injection pain

This is a lengthy procedure so always remember to offer the patient opportunities to get up and move, use the bathroom, or eat/drink when needed. Pay attention to the ergonomics of the patient and take care when positioning the patient so that they can be as comfortable as possible

KEEP IN MIND TIME AND POSITION

Intraoperative Patient Comfort Measures

LIST OF ITEMS PATIENT SHOULD BRING

Patients benefit from distraction from the procedure. They should be encouraged to bring headphones and prepare some music or favorite podcasts

Consider placing a TV up high where the patient can easily view while the grafts are being transplanted. Keep discrete trash receptacles with lids or built into cabinets so that bloody gauze and other items can be discarded and kept from the patient's vision

SET UP OF PATIENT ROOM

INTUITIVE CARE

Surgeon and team should work to develop an intuition about which patients prefer to "zone out" and which would prefer to be engaged in conversation. Humor is a great distraction for many patients. Ensure that team conversations remain appropriate and avoid words like "opps" or "I'm sorry" that could be misinterpreted by the patient

Fig. 7. Intraoperative patient comfort measures.

donor harvesting sites twice daily for 4 to 5 days until they heal.[46]

Graft Placement

The patient is reclined in a comfortable supine position and 2 to 3 surgical assistants place grafts into the recipient sites using microvascular forceps. The surgeon observes the placement carefully and provides any necessary direction as the placement of the grafts is the most technically challenging part of the procedure. Hemostasis can be a challenge for some patients, but the bigger challenge is the "popping" of grafts out of the recipient site. If grafts are not staying in the follicle, gentle pressure should be applied with a saline-soaked cotton tipped applicator and held for 5 to 15 seconds. The team functions best when 2 assistants place grafts while 1 assistant rotates in when a break is needed.

Postoperative Protocol

An overnight nonstick dressing is applied to the patient's scalp. The patient is not likely to experience severe postoperative pain, but we recommend prescribing a small quantity of Tylenol #3 for use every 4 to 6 hours in the event of pain on the first day after the procedure. The patient also receives a prescription for prednisone 40 mg once daily for 3 days to minimize frontal edema. The patient is advised to begin regular activities immediately but avoid strenuous exercise. The

day after the procedure, the patient removes the bandage, showers, and allows water to run over the grafts. The patient should be cautioned against picking or rubbing the perifollicular crusts, and they should not allow their comb to touch the crusted areas when brushing their hair. Emollient application is applied daily to the donor area to help with secondary intention healing. Staples or sutures are removed on postoperative days 7 through 10, and during that time the perifollicular crust naturally resolves. Once suture removal is complete, the patient is permitted to resume their normal exercise program. The patient returns for follow-up between months 8 and 12. Most of the time, grafts enter the telogen phase for the first 3 months following transplantation before entering the anagen growth phase, so it is difficult or impossible to evaluate the success of the transplant procedure for nearly a year[48] (**Box 1**).

TREATMENT RESISTANCE/COMPLICATIONS

Surgical complications from hair transplantation occur rarely, developing in approximately 2% to 3% of patients and often much less with experienced teams. Folliculitis and pustules occasionally develop and require treatment with topical or oral antibiotics. Neurosensory complications, including neuralgias, prolonged pain sensations, pruritus, or numbness, occur infrequently and generally resolve on their own in days and almost always before the postoperative follow-up at 8 to

12 months. Very rarely, patients experience abnormal scarring or keloid formation in the donor or recipient sites. Some patients experience a temporary effluvium throughout their scalp, including the donor site. Aesthetic or efficacy complications are more likely than surgical complications. Overall, less than 85% to 90% growth and survival of the grafts is considered an unfavorable

outcome. Patient factors, including adherence to postoperative instructions, preoperative and postoperative medical management of hair loss, smoking history, presence of severe actinic damage, and the health and vascularity of the scalp play a role in the likelihood of treatment success. The patient requires long-term continued medical management for hair loss and may require future transplant procedures. In this sense, the clinical relationship between the patient and surgeon is often ongoing.[45,48]

NEW DEVELOPMENTS

FUE is now used for a variety of different indications, including transplantation of body hair, camouflage of scars, and in treating scarring alopecia. Transplantation of eyebrow hair, for example, can be transformative for the appearance of the patient. Transgender patients may pursue hair transplantation during their transition and a growing awareness of the specific needs of our transgender patient populations benefits our patients and can make a major impact on their lives. In treatment of scarring alopecia, it is vital to adequately treat the inflammation first and inform the patient of the potential for the inflammatory disease to recur on the scalp. Cultural competence is fortunately increasing in all areas of medicine, and hair transplantation is no different. In addition to considering variation in hair density, caliber, and common inflammatory dermatosis among patients of different ethnicities, an understanding of hair grooming and hair styling preferences among various ethnic groups is essential to competent and compassionate care of these patients. African American patients are more likely to develop traction alopecia and central centrifugal alopecia (CCCA) due to chronic tension on follicles from braiding or extensions as well as use of strong chemical relaxers. For these patients, control of inflammation with topical steroids, steroid injections, and/or oral doxycycline before transplant improves outcomes.

Improving graft survivability before implantation is a major goal and a variety of solutions have been proposed with modest or negligible results. Some surgeons use intraoperative PRP injections but we prefer postoperative PRP injections to the recipient area as a long-term strategy months after transplantation. Autologous plasma is used as the holding media for follicles during the procedure in some clinics, although it is unclear whether this improves graft survival.

The main limitation in meeting the patient's goals is the amount of donor hair available; thus, cloning of hair follicles will likely be the next major

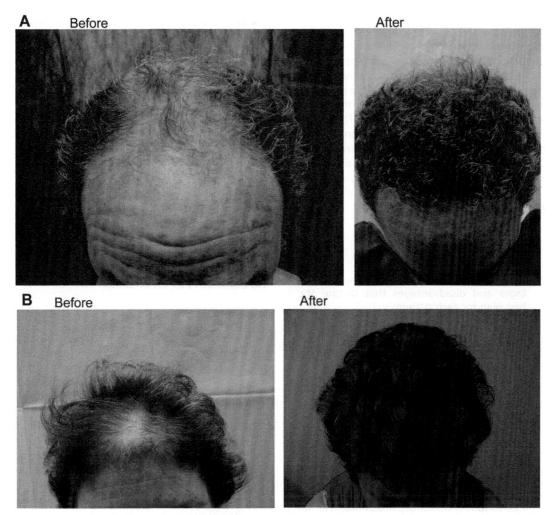

Fig. 8. Two patients before and after transplantation. (*A*) Male with androgenetic alopecia before and after transplant. (*B*) Female with androgenetic a;opecia before and after transplant.

revolutionary advancement in hair transplantation over the next decade or two. Numerous in vitro and animal model studies demonstrate the potential efficacy of replication of hair follicles, but the challenges of translation into a useable in vivo model are vast and application of this technology remains years away.[10,46]

EVALUATION OF OUTCOME AND LONG-TERM RECOMMENDATIONS

When the patient returns for the 8-month to 12-month postoperative appointment, photography is obtained and compared. A long-term medical management plan is created and reviewed with the patient, ideally including 2 hair loss treatments. The patients may choose which treatment modalities best fit their lifestyle and personal preferences. Topical minoxidil, oral finasteride, red light

therapy at home, and PRP injections are the most common maintenance treatments (**Fig. 8**).

SUMMARY

The principles and techniques of hair restoration were pioneered by dermatologists, and hair transplantation techniques involve solely cutaneous structures; therefore, these operative procedure are extraordinarily well-suited for integration into the practice of a dermatologic surgeon. Many dermatologists view initiation of a hair transplantation program with trepidation because of the long learning curve required for both the surgeon and the entire surgical team, and the need to dedicate a significant amount of clinic time and space to this procedure. In addition, some of the more modern equipment used in hair transplants, like the robotic unit, require a large investment. However, even with these initial challenges on implementation, hair transplantation is one of the most transformative and rewarding procedures that we can offer our patients. Few procedures combine a detailed technical procedure with an opportunity for artistic expression. It will be exciting to see the many ways in which innovative technologies further revolutionize our ability to replenish hair. The positive psychosocial impact of successful treatment of hair loss among patients leads to a very gratifying procedure for the surgeon and often a rewarding long-term doctor-patient relationship.

CLINICS CARE POINTS

- Both FUT and FUE techniques have advantages and disadvantages that dictate the best plan for each patient.
- A thorough patient evaluation is the first step to ensuring a successful hair transplant procedure. The surgeon must evaluate the patient's hair follicle density, average caliber of the hair shaft, pattern of alopecia, exacerbating hair loss factors, and predicted future pattern of hair loss in determining whether a patient is a candidate for transplant.
- Female patients in particular benefit from a more comprehensive hair loss work up and laboratory evaluation.
- Pharmacologic and medical management of hair loss with some combination of modalities including minoxidil, finasteride, PRP injections, or red light treatment should be initiated prior to transplant and continued long term.
- Hair transplantation is a lengthy and detailed procedure with a steep learning curve. Making a great transplant team requires practice and it is advisable to begin with smaller cases and progress towards larger cases (such as 1000 to 2500 grafts) with time.
- FUT can be used in patients with longer hair styles if the scalp has sufficient elasticity. A trichophytic closure of the strip minimizes scarring.
- FUE allows the surgeon to obtain a large number of grafts with little to no visible scarring using a 0.75mm to 1.2mm punch device.

Patient comfort measures are extremely important during the lengthy FUE procedure.

- Hairline planning requires attention to detail and frank discussion with the patient, given the predicted pattern of future hair loss.

- Puncture wounds of recipient sites are made using #19 or #20 gauge needles penetrating at a 30 to 45 degree angle that mimics normal hair growth.
- Motorized and robotic extraction devices increase the speed of the extraction process.
- Surgical assistants place grafts into recipient sites using microvascular forceps as the surgeon observes and directs.
- Postoperative care is important in the first ten days and patients need specific post-operative instructions day by day. Prednisone 40mg daily for three days helps prevent edema.
- Transplant success can not be entirely evaluated for a year or more.

DISCLOSURE

No disclosures for either author.

REFERENCES

1. International Society of Hair Restoration Surgery. Practice Census Results. 2020: Accessed online https://ishrs.org/wp-content/uploads/2020/05/Report-2020-ISHRS-Practice-Census-05-22-20.pdf.
2. Hadshiew IM, Foitzik K, Arck PC, et al. Burden of hair loss: stress and the underestimated psychosocial impact of telogen effluvium and androgenetic alopecia. J Invest Dermatol 2004;123:455–7.
3. Cash TF. The psychosocial consequences of androgenetic alopecia: a review of the research literature. Br J Dermatol 1999;141:398–405.
4. Sasagawa M. Hair transplantation. Jpn J Dermatol 1923;30:493.
5. Okuda H. The study of clinical experiments of hair transplantation. [in Japanese]. Jpn J Dermatol Urol 1939;46:1–11.
6. Orentreich N. Autografts in alopecias and other selected conditions. Ann N Y Acad Sci 1959;83:463.
7. Uebel CO. Micrografts and minigrafts: a new approach for baldness surgery. Ann Plast Surg 1991;27(5):476–87.
8. Shiell RC. A review of modern surgical hair restoration techniques. J Cutan Aesthet Surg 2008;1(1):12–6.
9. Paus R, Cotsarelis G. The biology of hair follicles. N Engl J Med 1999;341:491–7.
10. Sharma R, Ranjan A. Follicular unit extraction (FUE) hair transplant: curves ahead. J Maxillofac Oral Surg 2019;18(4):509–51.
11. Limmer BL. Elliptical donor stereoscopically assisted micrografting as an approach to further refinement in hair transplantation. J Dermatol Surg Oncol 1994;20:789–93.
12. Rassman WR, Bernstein RM, McClellan R, et al. Follicular unit extraction: minimally invasive surgery for hair transplantation. Dermatol Surg 2002;28(8):720–8.

13. Blume-Peytavi U, Blumeyer A, Tosti A, et al. Guidelines for diagnostic evaluation in androgenetic alopecia in men, women and adolescents. Br J Dermatol 2011;164(1):5–15, 6.

14. Gupta M, Mysore V. Classifications of patterned hair loss, a review. J Cutan Aesthet Surg 2010;9(1):3–12.

15. Vogel JE. Hair transplantation in women: a practical new classification system and review of technique. Aesthet Surg J 2002;22(3):247–59.

16. Chartier MB, Hoss DM, Grant-Kels JM. Approach to the adult female patient with diffuse nonscarring alopecia. J Am Acad Dermatol 2002;47:809–18.

17. Rebora A, Guarrera M, Baldari M, et al. Distinguishing androgenetic alopecia from chronic telogen effluvium when associated in the same patient. Arch Dermatol 2005;141:1243–5.

18. Kantor J, Kessler LJ, Brooks DG, et al. Decreased serum ferritin is associated with alopecia in women. J Invest Dermatol 2003;121:985–8.

19. Harries MJ, Trueb RM, Tosti A, et al. How not to get scar(r)ed: pointers to the correct diagnosis in patients with suspected primary cicatricial alopecia. Br J Dermatol 2009;160:482–501.

20. Hillmer A, Hanneken S, Ritzmann S, et al. Genetic variation in the human androgen receptor gene is the major determinant of common early onset androgenetic alopecia. Am J Hum Genet 2005;77:140–8.

21. Levy-Nissenbaum E, Bar-Natan M, Pras E. Confirmation of the association between male pattern baldness and the androgen receptor gene. Eur J Dermatol 2005;15(5):339–40.

22. Dinh Q, Sinclair R. Female pattern hair loss: current treatment concepts. Clin Interv Aging 2007;2(2):189–99.

23. Hillmann K, Blume-Peytavi U. Diagnosis of hair disorders. Semin Cutan Med Surg 2009;28:33–8.

24. Ludwig E. Classification of the types of androgenetic alopecia (common baldness) occurring in the females sex. Br J Dermatol 1977;97:247–54.

25. Norwood OT. Male pattern baldness: classification and incidence. South. Med J 1975;68:1359–65.

26. Olsen EA, Whiting D, Bergfeld W, et al. A multicenter, randomized, placebo-controlled double-blind clinical trial of a novel formulation of 5% topical minoxidil foam vs placebo in the treatment of androgenetic alopecia in men. J Am Acad Dermatol 2007;57:767–74.

27. Messenger AG, Rundegren J. Minoxidil: mechanisms of action on hair growth. Br J Dermatol 2004;150:186–94.

28. Avram MR, Cole JP, Gamndelman M, et al. The potential role of minoxidil in the hair transplantation setting: roundtable consensus meeting of the 9th annual meeting of the International Society of Hair Restoration Surgery. Dermatol Surg 2002;28:894–900.

29. Mella JM, Perret MC, Manzotti M, et al. Efficacy and safety of finasteride therapy for androgenetic alopecia: a systematic review. Arch Dermatol 2010;146:1141–50.

30. Price V, Roberts J, Hordinsky M, et al. Lack of efficacy of finasteride in postmenopausal women with androgenetic alopecia. J Am Acad Dermatol 2000;43:768–76.

31. Rogers N, Avram M. Pharmacotherapy. In: Unger W, Shapiro R, Unger M, et al, editors. Hair transplantation. 5th edition. London: Informa Healthcare; 2010. p. 91–101.

32. Sato A, Takeda A. Evaluation of efficacy and safety of finasteride 1 mg in 3177 Japanese men with androgenetic alopecia. J Dermatol 2012;39(1):27–32.

33. Redman HW, Tangen CM, Goodman PJ, et al. Finasteride does not increase the risk of high-grade prostate cancer: a bias-adjusted modeling approach. Cancer Prev Res 2008;1:174–81.

34. D'Amico AV, Roehrborn CH. Effect of 1mg/day finasteride on concentrations of serum prostate-specific antigen in men with androgenetic alopecia: a randomized controlled trial. Lancet Oncol 2007;8:21–5.

35. Overstreet JS, Fug VL, Gould J, et al. Chronic treatment with finasteride daily does not affect spermatogenesis or semen production in young men. J Urol 1999;162:1295–300.

36. Iorizzo M, Vincenzi C, Voudouris S, et al. Finasteride treatment of female pattern hair loss. Arch Dermatol 2006;142:298–302.

37. Fun HC, Kwon OS, Yeon JH, et al. Efficacy, safety, and tolerability of dutasteride 0.5mg once daily in male patients with male pattern hair loss: a randomized, double blind, placebo controlled phase III study. J Am Acad Dermatol 2010;63:252–8.

38. Avram MR, Rogers NE. The use of low-level light for hair growth. J Cosmet Laser Ther 2009;11(2):110–7.

39. Uebel CO, da Silva JB, Cantarelli D, et al. The role of platelet plasma growth factors in male pattern baldness surgery. Plast Reconstr Surg 2006;118(6):1458–66 [discussion: 1467].

40. Avram M, Rogers N. Contemporary hair transplantation. Dermatol Surg 2009;35(11):1705–19.

41. Marzola M. Single-scar harvesting technique. In: Haber R, Stough DB editors. Hair transplantation. Elsevier; 2006;p. 83–6.

42. Mayer ML. Scalp elasticity measurement. Hair Transpl Forum 2005;4:122.

43. Marzola M. Trichophytic closure of the donor area. Hair Transpl Forum Int 2005;15:113–6.

44. Dua A, Dua K. Follicular unit extraction transplant. J Cutan Aesthet Surg 2010;3(2):76–81.

45. Shapiro R. Principles and techniques used to create a natural hairline in surgical hair restoration. Facial Plast Surg Clin North Am 2004;12:201–17.

46. Vogel JE, Jimenez F, Cole J, et al. Hair restoration surgery: the state of the art. Aesthet Surg J 2012; 33(1):128–51.

47. Avram MR, Watkins SA. Robotic follicular unit extraction in hair transplantation. Dermatol Surg 2014; 40(12):1319–27.

48. Avram MR, Rogers N, Watkins S. Side effects from follicular unit extraction in hair transplantation. J Cutan Aesthet Surg 2014;27(3):177–9.

Combination Approaches for Combatting Hair Loss

Paul T. Rose, MD, FISHRS, JD

KEYWORDS

- Androgenetic alopecia • Follicular unit transplantation • Follicular unit excision
- Platelet rich plasma (PRP) • Scalp micropigmentation • Minoxidil • Finasteride

KEY POINTS

- Multiple treatment modalities exist to treat hair loss. These can include various medications as well as surgical procedures.
- While surgery is often the approach for androgenetic alopecia the process is often limited by the amount of donor hair available.
- By combining surgical procedures with medication treatment and camouflage techniques the patient may be able to achieve the optimal cosmetic result.

INTRODUCTION

Many men, women, and children suffer from hair loss. The cause may be genetic, or it may be due to other factors such as metabolic disorders, trauma, or inflammatory or non-inflammatory dermatologic diseases.

The most common form of hair loss is androgenetic alopecia. For these patients the clinician has multiple strategies available to try to restore the hair that has been lost. When dealing with limited donor hair the patient may want to consider medical and surgical treatments to attempt to provide adequate coverage.

MEDICAL THERAPY
Minoxidil

Minoxidil has been commercially available for androgenetic alopecia since the late 1980s. It was originally used for hypertension, and a side effect of hirsutism was noted.[1] This led to use for hair loss in men and women.

The mechanism of action of minoxidil[2] has not been fully elucidated. It is believed that it has an effect on potassium channels. The fact that it does cause vasodilatation does not seem directly related to the positive action on hair growth moving hair into the anagen phase of the hair cycle.[3,4]

Minoxidil is usually provided in the liquid or foam form, and the usual concentration is 5%. It can be combined with other medications such as a steroid and retinoic acid. A 2% version is available for women but most clinicians advise female patients to use the stronger concentration unless there are adverse reactions with the stronger formulation.

In some instances, minoxidil can be prescribed as an oral medication. We start at a dose of 1.25 mg per day and work up to a higher dose of 2.5 mg if the patient is not having any adverse reaction such as hypotension, edema, and excess hair growth in areas where hair growth is not desired.

Finasteride and Dutasteride

For almost all male patients, unless there is a contraindication, we will suggest that the patient consider taking finasteride 1 mg per day.[4,5] If the patient has any side effects we consider lowering the dose to 1 mg every other day.

Unfortunately, many patients are reluctant to take this medication due to fears of change in libido and/or erectile dysfunction.[6] Recent studies have shown that such a reaction is very rare, and it does not seem to be permanent if the drug is stopped. Contradictory material in the literature suggests that there is a permanent effect related to libido and erectile function but again this is

Miami Skin and Hair Institute, 4425 Ponce de Leon Boulevard, Suite 230, Coral Gables, FL 33146, USA
E-mail address: paultrose@yahoo.com

Dermatol Clin 39 (2021) 479–485
https://doi.org/10.1016/j.det.2021.04.004
0733-8635/21/© 2021 Elsevier Inc. All rights reserved.

disputed by most of the clinicians prescribing the drug.[7] Nevertheless, it may be plausible that there is a small segment of patients who are particularly sensitive to finasteride and could possibly have permanent changes. It should be noted that the reports and journal articles indicating permanent adverse effects often do not include adequate statistical analysis.

Finasteride may be considered for female pattern alopecia in women who are no longer of childbearing age or who are unable to become pregnant. Concern exists for the use of finasteride in women because it can cause fetal abnormalities.

The response to finasteride in women is variable, as there is a subset of women who may respond but it seems to be a small segment of the population.[8] It seems that female pattern is not as closely linked to dihydrotestosterone (DHT) as it is in male pattern alopecia.

Dutasteride is similar to finasteride in that it blocks the conversion of testosterone to dihydrotestosterone via the alpha-reductase pathway. Dutasteride works on both of the alpha reductase pathways leading to the conversion of testosterone to DHT.[4,9] There is concern that dutasteride is more likely to cause side effects, and there are reports that dutasteride can permanently lower sperm counts in some individuals taking the medication. Some clinicians suggest that the patient freeze sperm before starting the medication.

There does seem to be some correlation to exacerbation of depression in patients who have depression, and patients must be advised of this before going onto these medications. A proper psychological evaluation is suggested in such cases before prescribing the drug.

Spironolactone

Spironolactone possesses antiandrogen properties.[10] Many women have a history of polycystic ovaries, and spironolactone can help to lower androgens in these patients. Menopausal and postmenopausal patients may have elevated androgens that could contribute to hair loss.

Spironolactone can be used for women suffering hair loss. The starting dose is often 50 mg per day and increased to 100 mg BID if tolerated. Care must be taken to avoid hypokalemia. A baseline potassium level is advised.

LOW-LEVEL LIGHT LASERS

The use of low-level lasers/LEDs can also be prescribed to help patients slow down hair loss and perhaps regrow some hair.[11-15] There are a multitude of these devices on the market, and the efficacy is very similar to topical minoxidil. The mechanism of action seems to be through activation of cyclic AMP. These devices use a wavelength of approximately 635 to 650 nm, and the devices in many cases have been approved as safe under Food and Drug Administration 510(K) guidelines. Curiously the wavelengths for enhancing DNA production are outside of the aforementioned wavelength range.[14]

Platelet-Rich plasma

In the past few years the use of platelet-rich plasma (PRP) has been advocated for hair loss.[16,17] The platelets contain numerous growth factors and when activated the platelets release the factors. The factors seem to produce renewed hair growth. Initially there was a skeptical reaction to the possibility that PRP might benefit patients with androgenetic hair loss,[18] but more recent data strongly suggest a positive response with PRP.[19,20]

Interestingly, a recent journal article reported that although patients treated with PRP versus minoxidil actually had a better measured response to minoxidil over PRP, the patients subjectively felt that the PRP was more effective.[21]

It is important to note that although the term PRP is used to denote concentrated platelets, there are many different systems to produce PRP. The systems concentrate platelets to varying degrees and with varying amounts of leukocytes and erythrocytes. The author has tested multiple systems and found that at the time of testing some systems did not concentrate the platelets in spite of manufacturer's claims that the platelets were being concentrated.[22] The concentration of the platelets and amount of leukocytes may be important in determining the ability of the PRP to produce positive results.

The use of PRP seems to be quite safe. At times patients may experience a "burning sensation" for a short time after the procedure or perhaps a feeling of pruritus. There can be localized edema. A serious side effect has been reported involving an embolism that led to a stroke in a patient.[23]

The mechanism of delivery of the PRP may be a factor in efficacy. The author has found that injection depth should be at about the level of the bulb, and as the needle is withdrawn the material is placed in a retrograde manner along the follicle up to the area of the sebaceous glands.

Some physicians advocate a microneedling method of injection of PRP. Based on hair anatomy it would seem that microneedling is not the most advantageous way to deliver the PRP to the areas of the stem cells in the follicles.

Microneedling however by itself may induce a positive hair growth response apart from PRP.[24]

The trauma of microneedling may induce some of the factors associated with PRP, and the response of the skin to the needling may upregulate WNT gene, which is associated with increased hair growth.

It is unclear as to what the protocol for PRP should be for treating hair loss in an ongoing manner. The author suggests a treatment and then a waiting period of 1 to 2 months. If there is a response, another treatment is at about 3 months. If there is a positive response we suggest treatments 2 to 4 times per year. To measure response it is suggested that photographs be obtained of the areas treated and measurements of hair mass be acquired with a device such as the Hair Check (Iberius Inc, Miami, Florida, USA).

The injection of PRP into localized areas is typically performed by first using a local anesthetic to create a ring block to anesthetize the area of injection. We have found that providing nitrous oxide gas via a patient controlled system can make the procedure far less uncomfortable for patient. The use of a cooling device such as a Zimmer (Zimmer Medizin Systems, Irvine, California, USA) can also be helpful.

When performing hair transplant surgery we advise using the PRP for its wound healing properties in the area of donor harvesting and injecting PRP into the area of the recipient grafts. Placing it in the area of the grafts seems to improve graft survival, allow for more dense packing of grafts, and there seems to be a faster growth of the grafts.

For patients who have areas of scarring due to trauma or other forms of cicatricial alopecia that is "burned out" we find that using PRP before a hair transplant to be very beneficial. This is especially true in areas of atrophic skin. The PRP is given a month or two before surgery. At times we may suggest 2 treatments before surgery. At times the use of PRP and a matrix product such as Acell (Acell Inc, Columbia, MD, USA) can be used to try to enhance the PRP effect by possibly providing slower and longer release of growth factors.

The PRP aids in building up the skin, providing a better vasculature network and provides a more fertile environment in which to place the grafts; this seems to increase survivability and allows for closer placement of grafts.

Exosomes

Exosomes are vesicles derived from cells that contain genetic information and other cell products. They were originally thought to contain waste products of cells but we have learned that in fact they are an important means for cells to communicate with one another.[25]

The exosomes can be harvested from cell or made artificially. Materials such as drugs can be placed into them, and they are able to cross the blood-brain barrier.

There are reports of the use of exosomes derived from being used to try to induce hair regrowth. Studies in mice[26,27] have recently shown that exosomes derived from mice can induce hair growth by affecting β-catenin. There is a study looking at exosomes and human hair growth.

Stem Cells

Stem cells have been promoted as a possible means to generate new hair and restart hair growth in miniaturizing hair. Typically the cells are obtained from adipose cells or bone marrow cells and often times the preparation is combined with PRP.[28]

There are several myths about stem cells that pervade the news and other media. These include reports that stem cells "know where to go" and that stem cells "turn into the cells" of the tissue that they are deposited into.[29–31]

These stem cells are considered "multipotent," whereas the cells most able to evolve into any cell top are referred to as pluripotent. The cells most capable to develop into any type of cell are referred to as totipotent, and these cells are the cells that form in early embryogenesis forming the 3 embryonic layers, ectoderm, endoderm, and mesoderm.

The evidence is clear that new hairs do not develop from the stem cell preparations derived from abdominal fat or bone marrow that are then injected into the scalp. Rather the cells degrade and dissipate. As they do so there are signals sent out to other cells and growth factors that may promote regrowth of miniaturizing hairs.

Although it is true that there are ways to take an adult cell and dedifferentiate it, the process is not easy nor reliable. Most of the work on dedifferentiation has taken place in murine cells as opposed to human cells.

The author has used adipose derived stem cells with success but the effect is temporary and the process is expensive.

A recent study has demonstrated that cell-enriched autologous fat grafts that contain multipotent stem cells can assist in hair regrowth. The cell mixture apparently reactivated dormant hair follicles. The protocol has not been elucidated. The patients were followed-up for 1 year and continued to have a positive response from baseline but it is unknown as to whether the effects are long-lasting. Further studies are needed to ascertain if one treatment is sufficient or multiple procedures are required to sustain an effect.[32]

Atrophic Skin and Hair Restoration

As noted earlier, there are times when the patient's skin is atrophic and not ideal for transplantation. By using fat grafts that may also serendipitously contain stem cells there can be an improvement in the texture of the skin. There is an accompanying increase in vascularity, and this may make for a more suitable graft placement milieu.[32]

It has been found that using PRP can also aid in restoring a more normal skin thickness and vascular status. Such usage may allow for hair transplants into an area that might ordinarily be too thin to transplant into, and this is often the case with skin damaged by irradiation.

THE ASSESSMENT OF CHANGES IN HAIR GROWTH WITH THERAPIES

A crucial aspect to medical therapy is the assessment of the efficacy of treatment. Although photographic evidence can be helpful, just taking serial photographs often does not convey changes especially if they are subtle.

Methods exist to provide a more accurate evaluation of treatment of the patient and the physician. The Hair Check device (Iberius LLC, Miami, FL, USA) invented by Dr Bernard Cohen[33] based on the concept of hair mass discussed by Dr James Arnold years ago is a very precise way of determining the response to therapy. Other hair measurement devices that take enhanced photos or video also can be helpful.

The primary point is that in providing medical therapy there should be some objective measuring system to assess if the modalities selected are in fact aiding the patient.

Surgical Therapy

There are essentially 2 methods for obtaining hair grafts surgically. The more traditional method is to obtain a strip of hair bearing tissue and then dissect the strip down to individual follicular units (FUs). The FUs are the naturally occurring hair groupings. They generally exist as cluster of grouping of 1 to 4 hairs. Older methods use combined FUs to form mini-grafts with multiple FUs but this approach has largely been supplanted by the FU method, which is now termed follicular unit transplantation (FUT). Although there is no indication from the name that a strip is used the convention is to call this procedure FUT.[34,35]

The more recent method for performing hair transplantation is referred to as follicular unit excision (FUE).[36,37] As with strip harvesting FUs are used. They are, however, harvested individually with a handheld device with a punch attachment, which may be mechanized, or they can be harvested with a robotic device named the Artas system (Venus Concept, Toronto, Canada).[38,39]

There are many handheld devices currently available. Some of these devices can oscillate along with rotating and vibration. All these parameters can be adjusted to try to avoid transection of FU grafts and provide increased graft survival.

In all of the systems, including the purely manual method, a punch of various design is placed in the device, and it is used in the same manner as a dermatologic skin biopsy punch to try to capture intact FUs. In some instances the surgeon may elect to take a part of an FU. This can be done to further camouflage the donor harvest area and allow hairs to regrow within the individual FU harvest site. This technique is described as follicular isolation technique.[40]

Each technique has advantages and disadvantages. With the FUT method the surgeon is harvesting the best hair the patient will ever have. This is the hair just superior to the nuchal ridge, and it extends to the lateral aspects of the scalp, ending close to the insertion of the ears.

Oftentimes in patients with marked hair loss the surgeon can obtain more grafts than with FUE, assuming good skin laxity. In addition, the cost is usually significantly less than the FUE process. The disadvantage is that a linear scar is created, which may be evident depending on the length of hair of the patient. The FUT scar can be largely mitigated by using a trichophytic closure such as the "ledge closure."[41]

The advantage of FUE is that a linear scar is not created but round dotlike scars are nevertheless created, and if there is excess harvesting the donor area can be thinned out. If the patient wears his hair very short the "dots" created from the healed FUE wounds can be observed.

The cost for FUE is usually higher, and in most instances the patient has to shave the donor area for harvesting. Long hair FUE techniques are available, but the sessions are usually smaller, more tedious, and more expensive.

It is not uncommon for patients to undergo FUT procedures, and once the scalp laxity becomes limited the patient may switch to FUE procedure to obtain more donor hair. Similarly, FUE patients who reach a point where they can no longer have FUE may decide to switch to FUT procedures to expand the donor supply.

These techniques are covered more thoroughly in other chapters of this text.

Body hair

In cases where there is not enough scalp hair to perform an adequate session of transplants for a patient, body and beard hair can be used to supplement the donor hair available.[42]

Oftentimes a good source of hair is the chest area and the beard area. The disadvantage of the use of such hairs is that such hairs may not provide a good match in terms of hair caliber, curl, and other growth characteristics. Use of this hair is best when there is surrounding scalp hair to blend in with the body or beard hairs.

Also when the patient is seeking to add more hair to a region such as the beard the use of hair from the beard area such as under the chin can provide an optimal match in terms of hair caliber and growth characteristics.

The process for body hair harvesting requires the use of the FUE technique. When planning to use this method the patient should be on minoxidil topically for several weeks to encourage anagen growth. At approximately 1 week before surgery the patient is advised to shave the area, thus allowing the new hair growth to help differentiate the hairs into the anagen phase of hair development.[42]

A disadvantage to the use of body or beard hair is that the FUs are generally single hairs. On occasion some 2-hair groupings are found. In addition, the patient needs to be advised that the wounds created may heal as hypopigmented circular spots. There is also a general feeling that body hairs do not survive as well as scalp hairs.

Flaps, expansion, and scalp reduction surgery

In general the use of scalp reductions[43–48] and flaps[49] has fallen out of favor. Problems with scarring, stretch back of incisions, and altered hair direction has made the use of these techniques relatively obsolete.

However, in some cases, particularly trauma and cancer surgery cases where portions of hair bearing scalp are lost, the use of expanders and flaps can be life changing.[50,51] By using expanders existing areas of hair bearing tissue can be enlarged over several months to provide hair bearing skin that can then be moved into the areas without hair.

Patients must endure the discomfort of the actual expansion over several weeks to months, and having a large "balloon" on the head until the expansion is completed.

Scalp micropigmentation

Scalp micropigmentation is a relatively new modality available to enhance the results of hair transplantation or simply add to the visual appearance of hair in patients with thinning hair.[52,53] It is a method of tattooing the skin with inks that are used exclusively for this purpose. It is often performed by professionals who have experience performing tattooing for breast reconstruction of the nipple complex.

When done properly it appears as tiny dots that simulate the appearance of hair at the skin level. Some men who are not candidates for hair transplants may use this procedure exclusively to give the impression of having a shaved head with hair follicles still present. The technique seems to work ideally in areas where there is still some hair to further camouflage the area and make it appear more natural.

We find that it works exceptionally well in women where the hairline is retained and the remaining areas are diffusely thin. Although the hair transplantation may significantly improve the areas of hair loss there may be insufficient donor to fully cover the areas with transplanted hair.

SUMMARY

A significant portion of the adult population experiences hair loss. Children may experience hair loss but usually it is related to conditions that do not require surgery such as alopecia areata. At times children experience a physically traumatic event that results in hair loss.

There are several reasons for hair loss but in cases of androgenetic alopecia or inactive inflammatory hair loss disease, it may be possible to provide medical and or surgical therapy to regrow hair or maintain hair.

In all instances of using medical treatments it is imperative that the clinician try to impress on the patient the need for compliance, which can be very difficult, especially with male patients. Obviously the various medical treatments provide no benefit if they are not used.

In many instances there may not be enough hair to provide all the coverage that the patient desires. In such instances the physician has other possible modalities surgically and medically to try to fulfill the patient's request for the appearance of more hair.

By obtaining sufficient knowledge about the many resources that are available, whether surgical techniques or medical modalities, the physician can be a more competent hair loss clinician and provide optimal care for the patient.

CLINICS CARE POINTS

Pitfalls and Pearls

- It is imperative to avoid thinning out the donor area in FUE cases. It is generally safest to stay within the "safe zone'

- PRP varies with varying systems. It is unclear what the ideal protocol is for the treatment of hair loss
- The use of exosomes is currently unapproved by the FDA for the treatment of hair loss
- PRP can improve skin quality in cases where the skin is atrophic. This can allow a more "fertile" environment for grafts as vascularity is increased
- derived stem cells do not turn into new hairs. The cells die off and in so doing release cellular signals that promote regrowth or improved growth of hair follicles
- In using body hair as a donor it is suggested that the patient use Minoxidil 5% topically for approximately six weeks to push hairs into anagen. One week or so before surgery the area should be shaved to better visualize anagen hairs growing. These can then be harvested
- Body hair and beard hair can be used to improve the appearance of donor scars from FUT and FUE
- SMP is very useful for camouflaging donor scars
- Patients should be advised that scars are created whether one uses the FUT or FUE process. FUE scars a typically appear as hypo-pigmented dots.
- Oral minoxidil can be very helpful for hair loss but clinicians must be aware of possible side effects. It is advised to start with low doses and titrate upwards as needed.
- Low dose finasteride such as 0.5mg can be very effective for hair loss in males

DISCLOSURE

The author has received honoraria from the Eclipse Corporation for teaching PRP workshops.

REFERENCES

1. Zapacosta AR. Reversal of baldness in patient receiving minoxidil for hypertension. N Engl J Med 1980;287:1015–7.
2. Meisher ME, Cipkus LA, Taylor CJ. Mechanism of action of minoxidil sulfate induced vasodilatation: a role for increased K+ permeability. J Pharmacol Exp Ther 1988;245:751–60.
3. Olsen EA, Dunlap FE, Funicella T, et al. A randomized clinical trial of 5% topical minoxidil versus 2% topical minoxidil and placebo in the treatment of androgenetic alopecia in men. J Am Acad Dematol 2002;47(3):377–85.
4. Nusbaum AG, Rose PT, Nusbaum BP. Nonsurgical Therapy of Hair Loss. Facial Plast Surg Clin North Am 2013;21(3):335–42.
5. Kaufman KD, Olsen EA, Whiting D, et al. Finasteride in the treatment of men with androgenetic alopecia. Finasteride Male Pattern Hair Loss Study Group. J Am Acad Dermatol 1998;39(4 Part 1):578–89.
6. Traish AM, Hassan J, Guay AT, et al. Adverse side effects of 5 alpha reductase inhibition therapy persistent diminished libido and erectile dysfunction and depression in a subset of patients. J Sex Med 2011;8(3):872–84.
7. Haber R, Gupta AK, Epstein E. Finasteride for androgenetic is not associated with sexual dysfunction: a survey based, single centre, controlled study. J Eur Acad Dermatol Venereol 2019;33(7):1393–7.
8. Price VH, Roberts JL, Hordinsky M, et al. Lack of efficacy of finasteride in post-menopausal women with androgenetic alopecia. J Am Acad Dermatol 2000; 43(5 Part 1):768–76.
9. Eun HC, Kwon OS, Yeon JH, et al. Efficacy, safety, and tolerability of dutasteride).5 mg once daily in male patients with male pattern hair loss: a randomized mixed double blind placebo controlled phase III study. J Am Acad Dermatol 2010;63:252–8.
10. Sinclair R, Wewerinke M, Jolley D. Treatment of male pattern hair loss with oral anti-androgens. Br J Dermatol 2005;152(3):466–72.
11. Jimenez JJ, Wikramanayake TC, Bergfeld W, et al. Efficacy and safety of a low level laser device in the treatment of Male and Female Pattern Hair loss: a multicenter randomized Sham Device-controlled Double Blind study. Am J Clin Dermatol 2014;15(2):115–27.
12. Hamblin MR. Photobiomodulation for the management of alopecia, mechanisms of action, patient selection and perspectives. J Clin and Cosmetic and Investigational Dermatology 2006;(12):669–78.
13. Bernstein HF. Hair growth induced by diode laser treatment. Dermatol Surg 2005;31(5):584.
14. Keene S. The science of light bio-stimulation and low level laser therapy. Hair Transpl Forum Int 2014; 24(6):208–9.
15. Hamblin MR, Demidova TN. Mechanism of low level light therapy. Proc SPIE 2006;6140:1–12.
16. Uebel CO, Da Silva JB, Cantarelli D, et al. The role of platelet rich plasma in women with female androgenetic alopecia. Plast Reconstr Surg 2006;118(6): 1458–66.
17. Greco J, Brandt R. Preliminary experience and extended applications for the use of autologous platelet rich plasma in hair transplantation surgery. Hair Transpl Forum Int'l 2007;17(4):131–2.
18. Puig CJ, Reese R, Peters M. Double blind placebo controlled pilot study on the use of platelet rich plasma in women with female androgenetic alopecia. Dermatol Surg 2016;42(11):1243–7.
19. Heseler MJ, Shyam N. Platelet rich plasma and its utilities in alopecia, a systematic review. Dermatol Surg 2020;46(1):93–102.

20. Hausauer AK, Humphrey S. The physician guide to platelet rich plasma in Dermatologic Surgery part II, Clinical Evidence. Dermatol Surg 2020;46(4): 447–56.
21. Bruce AJ, Pincelli T, Heckman MG. A randomized controlled pilot trial comparing platelet rich plasma to topical minoxidil foam for treatment of androgenetic alopecia inn women. Dermatol Surg 2020; 46(6):820.
22. Rose PT, Nusbaum AG. A brief study examining the variability of PRP preparation systems. Hair Transpl Forum Int'l 2018;28(4):1–2.
23. Berti AF, Santillan A, Garcia-Currochano P. Acute stroke after scalp injection of platelet rich plasma and stem cells for hair loss. J Neurol Stroke 2015; 3(6):00112.
24. Dhurat R, Matthapatis S. Response of microneedling treatment in men with androgenetic alopecia who failed to respond to conventional therapy. Indian J Dermatol 2015;60(3):260–3.
25. Gurunathan S, Kang MH, Jeyaraj M, et al. Review of the isolation, characterization, biologic function and multifarious therapeutic approaches for exosomes. Cells 2019;8(4):307.
26. Rajendran RL, Gangadaran P, Bak SS, et al. Extracellular vesicles derived from MSCs activate dermal papilla cells in vitro and promotes hair follicle conversion from telogen to anagen in mice. Sci Rep 2017;7:11360.
27. Le Riche A, Aberdam E, Marchand L, et al. Extracellular vesicles from activated dermal fibroblast stimulate hair follicle growth through dermal papilla-secreted Norrin. Stem Cell 2019;37(9):1166–75.
28. Kuka G, Epstein J. Transplantation of cells enriched adipose tissue for follicular niche stimulation in early androgenetic alopecia: a multi center randomized blinded controlled investigation, the STYLE trial. Aest Surg J 2020;1–12.
29. Michler RE. Stem cell therapy for heart failure, methodist DeBakey. Cardiovasc J 2013;9(4):187–94.
30. Marks PW, Witten CM, Califf RM. Prospective- Clarifying stem cell therapy benefits and risks. N Engl J Med 2017;16:1007–9.
31. FDA warns about stem cell Therapies, consumer updates. Available at: http://www.fda.gov/consumers/consumer-update/fda-warns-about-stem-cell-therapies. Accessed September 3, 2019.
32. Kuka G, Epstein J, Aronowitiz J, et al. Cell enriched autologous fat grafts to follicular niche improves hair regrowth in early androgenetic alopecia. Aest Surg 2020;40(6):328–39.
33. Cohen B. The cross-section trichometer: a new device for measuring hair quantity, hair loss and hair growth. J Deratol Surg 2008;34(7):900–11.
34. Limmer BL. Elliptical donor stereoscopically assisted micro-grafting as an approach to further refinement in hair transplantation. Dermatol Surg 1994;20:789–92.
35. Bernstein RM, Rassman WR, Prose P, et al. Standardizing the classification and description of follicular unit transplantation and min-micrografting technique. Dermatol Surg 1998;24:957–63.
36. FUE Rassman WR, Bernstein RM, McCLellan JR, et al. Follicular unit extraction; minimally invasive surgery for hair transplantation. Dermatol Surg 2002;28:720–7.
37. Rassman WR, Harris JA, Bernstein RM. Follicular unit extraction. In: Stough D, Haber R, editors. Hair transplantation. Phila, PA: Elsevier Saunders; 2006. p. 133–7.
38. Harris JM. Robotic –assisted follicular unit extraction for hair restoration: case reports Cosmet. Dermaol 2012;25:284–7.
39. Rose PT, Nusbaum AG. Robotic Hair Transplantation. Dermatol Clin 2014;32(1):97–108.
40. Rose PT, Follicular Isolation technique, FIT, problems, solution and complications, Presentation Orlando Live Surgery Workshop, March 2-5, 2005, Orlando, Florida.
41. Rose PT. In: Unger W, Shapiro R, Unger R, editors. Ledge closure in Hair Transplantation fifth edition. New York: Informa Publishing; 2011. p. 281–4.
42. Umar S. The use of body hair and beard hair in hair restoration. Facial Plast Surg Clin North Am 2013;(30):469–77.
43. Alt TH. Scalp reductions as an adjunct to hair transplantation review of relevant literature and presentation of an improved technique. Dermatol Surg 1980; 6:1010–8.
44. Norwood OT, Shiell R, Morrison ID. Complication of Scalp Reduction. J Dermatol Surg Oncol 1983;9: 828–35.
45. Brandy DA. The bilateral occipital-parietal flap. J Dermatol Surg Oncol 1986;10:1062–6.
46. Brandy DA. Pitfalls and pearls of extensive scalp lifting. Am J Cosm Surg 1987;4(3):217–23.
47. Unger MH. In: Unger WP, Nordstrom REA, editors. Alopecia reduction in hair transplantation ed 2. NY, NY: Marcel Dekker, Inc; 1988. p. 435–518.
48. Rose PT. In: Moy RL, Lask G, editors. Scalp reductions in Principles and techniques in cutaneous surgery. New York: McGraw- Hill; 1996. p. 543–60.
49. Kabaker SS. Juri Flap procedure for the treatment of baldness; two year experience. Arch Otoloaryngol 1979;105(9):509–14.
50. Kabaker SS, Kridel RW, Krugman ME, et al. Tissue expansion in the treatment of alopecia. Arch Otolaryngol Head Neck Surg 1986;112(7):720–5.
51. Mangubat EA. Scalp repair using tissue expansion. Facial Plast Surg Clin North Am 2013;21(3):487–96.
52. Park JH, Mohs JS, Lee SY. Micro-pigmentation camouflaging scalp alopecia and scars in Korean patients. Aesthetic Plast Surg 2014;38(1):199–204.
53. Rassman WR, Pak JP, Kim J. Scalp micropigmentation a useful treatment for hair loss facial. Plast Surg Clinic North Am 2013;21(3):497–503.

Printed and bound by CPI Group (UK) Ltd, Croydon, CR0 4YY

03/10/2024

01040371-0009